GUIDE TO DRUG INFORMATION

PHOTO CREDITS

Front cover: Interior of the library of the royal monastery in Spain, El Escorial

Back cover: Interior of the Beinecke Library of Yale University

Inside covers: From the engraving by Cornelis Woudhanus of the chained library at Leyden University, 1610

GUIDE TO DRUG INFORMATION
by Winifred Sewell

HEALTH SCIENCE INFORMATION CONSULTANT

Currently Associated With

University of Maryland and

National Health Planning Information Center

Formerly With

National Library of Medicine,

Squibb Institute for Medical Research

Wellcome Research Laboratories

DRUG INTELLIGENCE PUBLICATIONS, INC., HAMILTON, ILL. 62341

COPYRIGHT © 1976 BY DRUG INTELLIGENCE PUBLICATIONS, INC.

All rights reserved

No part of this book may be reproduced

in any form without written

permission of the copyright holder

Library of Congress Catalog Number   75-17156
ISBN 0-914768-21-2

Printed in the United States of America by The Hamilton Press, Inc., Hamilton, Ill. 62341

PREFACE

During my whole professional life I have been concerned with one aspect or another of information transfer from the scientist or practitioner as the creator of knowledge to another scientist or practitioner as the user of knowledge. Only recently, however, have I been able to concentrate on facilitating the actual process of transfer. Studying this process has impressed me with the number of impediments which block it. One such impediment is the natural reluctance of the student or practitioner to learn techniques that are not obviously a part of his profession. When he gets to the library, he is concerned with the information he will find, not with the steps he will have to take to get it — he is concerned with the end, not the means. Yet he is blocked by problems ranging from lack of easy availability of materials to unfamiliarity with the increasingly complex secondary publications. The new on-line systems seem to make the student's life easier, but to get the most from them, he needs to understand even more elaborate rules than he has had to know to use manual systems efficiently.

Computer experts have adopted a jargon from which information scientists might borrow. They speak of a system as being "transparent" to the user, meaning that one can use it as though it were a clear window through which one sees without being aware of the glass. One gets the results of the computer process without knowing what happened to the transistors and drums. This is the ideal toward which I have devoted my efforts when working with information systems. The student, scientist, or practitioner should be able to get everything he needs by simply asking for it in straightforward language.

In that sense this book is only a stopgap, something to be used until the whole information transfer system becomes so transparent that it is not necessary to know anything about it to use it. But I am afraid the ideal is still a long way off. Until then the ultimate user will not get the most out of the system without becoming himself a part of it, not just as creator and consumer of knowledge, but also as a facilitator of his own information transfer process. The more he knows about techniques of using the literature, the more effective he will be.

That is the reason for the existence of this book. The kind of publication it is had additional influences. When Bill Woods asked me to write it five years ago, I questioned the need for yet another bibliography of the literature. There already existed several excellent ones. But it happened that just at that time I was beginning to work with undergraduates in pharmacy to teach them what I thought they should know about bibliography and the literature of pharmacy. I knew that the role of the pharmacist was changing and I soon learned that a great deal of change was also taking place in his education. As in other fields, it has become increasingly important to know how to find facts as well as to remember them and how to continue to learn as well as to learn at the moment. What is taught must also be relevant to the student's perceived needs. While recognition of the relevancy of literature use to pharmacy is not yet universal, the student is beginning to understand that he will be more and more dependent on reading throughout his career.

As the third-year students began to teach me what they didn't know, it became apparent that there was a mismatch between the existing guides and the student with no library background or at most an elementary lecture or two on how to use the library. The students did not need a booklist so much as a laboratory manual or cookbook that would tell them precisely how to find what they needed when they needed it. That is what I have tried to make this *Guide*. The students also showed me that they did not always know when they needed basic information. Much that is included here is not what I have been asked for, but what I have observed is lacking in the student's knowledge. In the light of his interest in ends, not means, the student may not wish to read this book straight through. Initially he should scan it closely enough to learn what it contains. When he does have a need, I hope he will find the answer here.

Because of its problem-solving orientation, the *Guide* may also be useful to people who have left their student days. I hope they will not object to its didacticism.

Over the years, a number of people have been involved with this book. Colleagues too numerous to mention have advised me about specific aspects. Two who made major contributions in its early stages are Marie Dickerman and Jeannine Garland. I am deeply grateful for their help. More recently, Don and Gloria Francke have spurred me on and given me counsel in finishing it. Most particularly, to the late Bill Woods go my thanks for encouraging the beginning and my regrets that he cannot see the conclusion.

October 1975 WINIFRED SEWELL

CONTENTS

CHAPTER	PAGE
Preface	v

PART 1

1 Introduction — 1

2 Drug Handbooks Introduction — 4

3 Looking at the Question — 6

4 Looking at the Handbook — 19
 Purposes of Handbooks—Scope and Coverage—Kind of Drug—Kind of Name—Special Features—Format Aspects

5 Choosing a Personal Collection — 38
 Annuals—Supplements to Annuals—Looseleaf Services—Card Services

PART 2

6 Primary Sources Introduction — 45

7 Periodicals — 57
 How to Find Periodical Titles of Interest

8 Books — 67
 Books on Pharmacy—Books on Pharmacology and Related Subjects—Books on Toxicology and Associated Disciplines—Drug Abuse Materials—Books on Medicine—Books on Chemistry

9 Other Primary Sources — 84
 Manufacturers' Literature—Patents—Government Documents—Theses and Research Studies

10 Directories, Dictionaries, Equipment Catalogs, and Other Reference Sources — 92

PART 3

11 Going Beyond One's Own Collection — 96
The Library—The Collection—Organization of the Collection—The Catalog

12 The Search — 104
Level of Effort—Organization of Work—Selection and Use of Literature Sources (Search Strategy)—Evaluation of the Search (Quality Control)

13 Secondary Services — 112
International Pharmaceutical Abstracts—Other Secondary Services in Pharmacy—*Chemical Abstracts*—*Current Abstracts of Chemistry* and *Index Chemicus*—*Index Medicus* and MEDLARS—*Excerpta Medica*—*Abstracts of World Medicine*—*Biological Abstracts* and *Bioresearch Index*—Other Secondary Services in Biology

14 Other Secondary Services — 144
An Index with a Different Approach—*Science Citation Index*—Indexes to Special Materials—Special Subjects—Unexpected Sources—Highly Specialized Sources—*FDA Clinical Experience Abstracts*—de Haen Services—Iowa Service—Derwent Services (*RingDoc* and Others)

15 Reviews and Encyclopedic Treatises — 152

16 Resources Beyond the Local Library — 156
Getting the Original Publication—Translations—Networks and Computer Services—Regional Medical Library Network—Commercial or University Centers—Individual Secondary Services—On-Line Services—Costs

PART 4

17 The Future — 164

18 Current Technology — 165
Computers—Input/Output Equipment—Microphotography and Photographic Transmission—Audiovisual Resources

19 Future Technology — 175

20 Keeping Up with the Literature During Technology Advances — 177
Organization—Cooperation—Standardization

21 Conclusion — 191

Index — 193

GUIDE TO
DRUG INFORMATION

CHAPTER *1*

PART 1

INTRODUCTION

⊓⊔⊓⊔⊓⊔⊓⊔⊓⊔⊓⊔⊓⊔⊓⊔⊓⊔⊓⊔⊓⊔⊓⊔⊓⊔⊓⊔⊓⊔

This book is intended to guide the pharmacist or other health professional in his use of the literature throughout a professional career that will encompass changes in basic therapeutic concepts, replacement of many of today's familiar drugs, development of new modes of communication, and major readjustments in the social and scientific role of the pharmacist himself. It is directed primarily to students. Yet it is written by a librarian-bibliographer who turned her attention to the drug field at the time of the introduction of penicillin.

My primary focus is the pharmacist because he is the one health professional involved with all aspects of drugs, and because thinking of pharmacy students I have known has helped me to keep the book practical. However, students with more limited interests in pharmaceuticals can benefit from it also. I would encourage them to translate the word "pharmacist" to "nurse," "physician," etc. as they feel it is appropriate.

Because of its audience and its purpose, we have decided against presenting a traditional bibliography, and have steadfastly resisted the temptation to list all possible sources on any given subject. Inevitably, because it is selective, it represents the author's prejudices and points of view. The selection of books is a display of old and new friends, with no guarantee that they are any better than some that have been omitted. Specific editions listed will be out of date almost before the student has learned their names, and in those volumes that survive, later editions will show changes in content and presentation to adjust to newer needs and the capabilities of newer publishing and communications equipment.

Since they are so transitory, we have attempted to list only a few helpful sources. We are devoting considerable space to the questions those sources will answer and the attributes of each that one should know to use them most effectively. By implication, we are saying that if you check these same attributes in new books and editions which you encounter, you will be able to select them judiciously and to use them effectively. In short, the methodology you use in selecting and evaluating reference sources can last a lifetime, while the sources themselves will be discarded and replaced like old clothes.

Behind the methodology described throughout this book is a three-pronged philosophy, which can be summarized as follows:

1. The literature is a tool just as surely as is a spectrograph or a microscope. As man's knowledge increases, he must rely more and more on its record, whether this be in his own book, a library, or a computerized data bank. To the pharmacist, literature is becoming a particularly important tool because of his increasing role as a consultant on drugs and their use. Indeed he is needed as a consultant because information on drugs and their actions has increased to the point that no single health scientist can carry in his mind all available drug knowledge at any one time, and the physician, nurse and other health professionals have become increasingly dependent on a specialist in pharmaceutical sciences.

2. A tool is as good as its user. Recently a graduate student admitted to being unaware that there was a synonym index at the back of *Merck Index*. The ignorance of this fact made his use of *Merck* only 25 percent effective because the back index contains about 42,000 names for the 10,000 individual substances, each listed under only one name in the body of the book.

3. A professional is constantly improving his tools and his techniques in their use. For this reason, the fourth section of this book will discuss the kinds of publication and data handling we may expect in the future and will suggest methods or habits

that will help you to keep up with the new information that will be generated during your professional career.

Part I of the book will deal intensively with a relatively few handbooks, many of which will be in the pharmacist's private collection, and with methods by which he can extract the most from them. Part 2 will describe periodicals, books, and other primary publications from which the pharmacist will select some he will wish to own and others he will consult in libraries. Part 3 will suggest resources that are available in libraries and elsewhere as guides to further information, and as already noted, Part 4 will discuss methods or habits that will help to absorb the new information and take advantage of new information-handling technology as it becomes available.

CHAPTER 2

DRUG HANDBOOKS
INTRODUCTION

⎍⎍⎍⎍⎍⎍⎍⎍⎍⎍⎍⎍⎍⎍⎍⎍⎍⎍⎍⎍⎍⎍⎍⎍⎍⎍

At the core of pharmacy is the drug, the substance which is the pharmacist's major concern, whether he is procuring it, dispensing it, or consulting with a doctor or patient about its use. And at the core of the pharmaceutical literature is the drug handbook. Such handbooks have also been called "drug information sources" or "drug compendia." We have chosen the word "handbook" because it seems best to describe the fact that we are talking about ready reference tools, books which will not be read cover to cover but which will be consulted frequently for specific items of information — books to be kept close at hand! Each gives a variety of information on a substantial number of individual drugs in a major section of the volume. While extensive information can be found in other important sources, they are included in later chapters because they are primarily general texts, such as *Goodman and Gilman*, to be read cover to cover, or they are mainly devoted to a very specific subject, such as Meyler's *Side Effects of Drugs*. There are, of course, no absolutes. Meyler will be used frequently as a handbook and *AMA Drug Evaluations* — included here among handbooks — may very well be a text in some courses.

Although there has been much discussion of a universal drug compendium (see for instance "Symposium on a New Drug Compendium, Why? What? How? When?" *Drug Information Bulletin,* 4:115-225, July-December 1970), there is as yet no one source that will answer all of a single user's questions. The reasons why there is no universal compendium are complex, but they can be summarized as follows:

1. There are a variety of purposes for a compendium or handbook — to provide standards, to provide means for identifying drugs, to provide information on actions and uses, and many more.

2. There are a variety of audiences to which handbooks are directed. The needs of community pharmacists, hospital pharmacists, and physicians are all better satisfied by some texts than by others, and the needs of each vary from time to time as they perform different roles.

3. There is a large number of drug products available in the United States and in other parts of the world, and there is a wide variety of uses to which they are put.

4. There is a large number of drug names, and they are of several different kinds.

The complexity of the sources leads to a dichotomy between the expert, who regards as an art his precision in using exactly the right source first, and the nonexpert user of the sources, who approaches them simplistically and assumes that there is no answer if he does not find it the first place he looks. There is no subtle art in using the sources if one analyzes carefully the thought processes of the expert in determining the right source at the right time. But it is tedious for the nonexpert to learn all of the essential information about each source, and it is ridiculous for him to attempt it. To bridge the gap, I have provided several tables that will enable you to compare sources in relation to your needs. I hope they will also help you to analyze your questions in terms of sources not on the list.

CHAPTER 3

LOOKING AT THE QUESTION

Since handbooks are intended to provide answers to questions, Table 1 categorizes the kinds of questions that can be answered. Generally speaking, one will turn to drug handbooks for specific facts about a drug and look further for more detailed discussions. To be specific, let's assume a hypothetical drug, *Farmlit,* and discuss some of the questions that can be answered by using the categorization in Table 1.

What is Farmlit? What other name is it marketed under? (Equivalent Identification)

All of the sources marked with a plus in the Equivalent Identification column will, at a minimum, give you another name for the drug. To find details of the kind of name provided, it will be necessary to use Table 2 as well.

Incidentally, the handbooks cannot solve for you the problem of interpreting a name in a garbled phone message or illegible prescription, but Benjamin Teplitsky has supplied a list of "look-alikes" and "sound-alikes" (*Pharmacy Times* 38:29-31, May 1972).

Where can I get Farmlit, in what forms, and at what cost? (Manufacturer; Market Availability; Prices)

The second, third, and fourth columns indicate which handbooks will contain answers. Since the three kinds of information are closely related, those sources which have pluses in all three columns are likely to be the best for any of these questions. One of the handbooks, *Facts and Comparisons,* does not actually give a wholesale or retail price. Instead, it provides a price index, so that a physician can tell which drug is cheaper for an equivalent effect in his patient. Some of the monographs in *Medical Letter* also mention equivalent prices of drugs.

Can I use Farmlit for a person in hepatic coma? My patient has developed a rash; could it be due to Farmlit? What is the maximum safe dose of Farmlit? What is the antidote for poisoning by Farmlit? Is it all right to prescribe Farmlit when the patient is also receiving insulin? Can I use it in an IV solution? (Adverse Reactions & Toxicity; Toxicology: Physical Incompatibilities)

In Table 1, we have isolated two general kinds of information on unintended or toxic reactions in line with the kinds of question one might need to answer.

Adverse Reactions & Toxicity (including side effects, interactions, and contraindications). Among side effects we include any unintended response to a drug, be it beneficial or adverse. The vast majority of side effects reported in drug handbooks are adverse ones, and some sources run the gamut from headache and nausea to liver damage under the terms "side effects" or "adverse reactions," so that it is fruitless to try to make a fine distinction among types. What is not given in most handbooks is any indication as to the incidence of serious toxicity.

Toxicology (including poisoning, antidotes, and animal toxicity). When quantitative information is encountered, it generally falls into the area of overdose levels in poisoning or of acute or chronic toxicity levels in animals. For this reason, those sources which give such quantitative information are identified separately on the table. Some of them, such as Clarke's *Isolation and Identification of Drugs,* also include antidotes for poisoning by many of the listed substances. When using the handbooks for toxicity information, we should remember that there are a number of texts and handbooks specifically on adverse reactions and poisoning to which one might better turn first. When dealing with poisoning from a more unusual substance, one should go to the handbook with the most extensive

Table 2. Editorial Aspects of Drug Handbooks

NAME	AUTHORITY	PURPOSE	GENERAL SCOPE
Accepted Dental Therapeutics	American Dental Association Council on Dental Therapeutics	To provide dentists with drug information needed in practice	All current U.S. drugs approved by Council, plus some not approved
AMA Drug Evaluations	American Medical Association Department of Drugs	To provide objective evaluations of drugs in relation to their uses	Major emphasis on drugs in official compendia, single entities introduced in past 10 years and products commonly prescribed
American Drug Index	Commercial	To provide a dictionary of different kinds of names for drugs	Same as purpose
American Hospital Formulary Service	American Society of Hospital Pharmacists	To provide monographs suitable for standards for hospital formularies	Selected drugs, and dentifrices, ointments, etc., that would be used in hospitals
Blue Book, American Druggist	Commercial	To provide a concise and complete source of information on availability, form, package, and prices of marketed drugs	All nationally and many locally distributed drug products
Compendium of Pharmaceuticals and Specialties	Canadian Pharmaceutical Association	". . . to present unbiased, factual information on drugs . . ."	All Canadian drugs not registered for sale to public for automedication
Current Drug Handbook	Commercial	To provide a concise source of drug information for nurses for quick reference	About 1,500 selected drugs
de Haen Nonproprietary Name Index	Commercial	To trace development of drugs since 1941	All single entities introduced in U.S. from 1941 to date, and in England, France, Germany, Italy, and Japan, 1969 to date
Dispensatory (U.S.)	Commercial, but published since 1833	To provide comprehensive information on drugs and chemicals in common use	Drugs, drug groups and chemicals, not necessarily currently marketed in U.S.
Drugs of Choice	Commercial	To provide a selection of drugs preferred for use in various diseases	Only those drugs which chapter editors choose to discuss; fairly comprehensive

Table 2. Editorial Aspects of Drug Handbooks

TYPE OF DRUG	TYPE OF NAME	COVERAGE BY: COUNTRY	TIME	SPECIAL FEATURES
Legend and non-legend	Generic and trade	U.S.	Currently marketed	Sections on dental formulas, therapeutics, and indexes of unaccepted drugs and monographs published in the *Journal of the American Dental Association*
Primarily legend	Generic and trade	U.S.	Currently marketed	Good introduction including concise section on drug interactions and description of official and regulatory bodies; pediatric dosage table is at back.
Legend and non-legend	Generic, trade, and chemical	U.S.	Current	Combinations listed under their ingredients
Primarily legend	Generic and trade	U.S.	Currently available	Definitions of terms for dosage forms at front. Appendixes on prescription writing, conversion tables, and biochemical tables
Legend and non-legend	Trade, if available; otherwise generic	U.S.	Currently marketed	Each issue has different features: for example, checklist for processing 3rd party claims in 1972 and description of a medical profile system in 1971
Primarily legend	Generic and trade	Canadian	Currently marketed	Also available in French. Appendix lists Canadian regulations, Canadian poison control centers, pediatric dosage, and conversion tables
Primarily legend	Generic and trade	U.S.	Currently used	Complete text is tabular in 6 columns: Name, Dosage and Administration, Uses, Action and Fate, Side Effects and Contraindications, and Remarks
Primarily legend	Generic and trade	US., Europe, and Japan	1941 to date including deletions	Year of introduction of each drug. Manufacturers' listing shows some mergers
Single-entity ingredients, legend and non-legend	Generic and common with trade synonyms	U.S.	Current and recent past	Drug class discussions for 20 different groups. Various salts and esters are grouped with bases or acids. The 26th edition dropped botanical descriptions and explanations of physical and chemical tests and assays, for which one must still use the 25th edition
Primarily legend	Generic and trade	U.S.	Current	New editions have new editors for some chapters so that viewpoints may change. 54 tables include childrens' doses and adverse reactions. Special drug index relates generic and trade names

Table 2. Editorial Aspects of Drug Handbooks

NAME	AUTHORITY	PURPOSE	GENERAL SCOPE
Drugs in Current Use	Commercial	To provide a quick reference tool on common drugs and more details on new drugs	Individual drugs likely to be used in general practice
Extra Pharmacopoeia	Council of Pharmaceutical Society of Great Britain	To give concise information on drugs in use worldwide	All drugs and constituents currently available in United Kingdom plus many used elsewhere
Facts and Comparisons	Commercial	To provide a comprehensive list of U.S. drugs with price comparisons of like drugs for physicians	Includes some deleted drugs plus all currently marketed
Handbook of Non-Prescription Drugs	American Pharmaceutical Association	To provide a comprehensive list of over-the-counter drugs and sundries	Includes dental preparations, hair preparations, etc., as well as nonprescription drugs for which composition is available
Identification Guide	Commercial	To make it possible to identify a tablet or capsule without the bottle or label	All Canadian products made available to the authors
Index Nominum	Société Suisse de Pharmacie	To provide basic information and worldwide synonyms for drugs	Single chemical entities in clinical use or on trial
International Nonproprietary Names	World Health Organization	To provide a generic name for a single entity that will be used internationally	Name, chemical name, and molecular formula for drugs with recommended names
International Pharmacopeia	World Health Organization	To provide standards of quality for adoption by any country	Physical and assay standards of selected drugs
Isolation and Identification of Drugs	Department of Pharmaceutical Sciences, Pharmaceutical Society of Great Britain	To provide isolation and identification information with particular reference to toxicology	Includes pesticides, chemicals, and other potentially toxic agents as well as drugs
Medical Letter	Commercial	To provide objective evaluation of drugs	Selects for review relatively new drugs and therapeutic devices, some investigational

Table 2. Editorial Aspects of Drug Handbooks

TYPE OF DRUG	COVERAGE BY:			SPECIAL FEATURES
	TYPE OF NAME	COUNTRY	TIME	
Primarily legend	Generic and some trade	U.S.	Current	Two parts, originally two books, entitled *Drugs in Current Use* and *New Drugs*. The latter was and continues to be much more complete
Legend, non-legend, and combinations	Generic, trade, and chemical	International	Current use somewhere, hence some old	Geographic information for many drugs. Separate lists of ancillary drugs and "counter proprietaries." Tables of abbreviations, weights and measures, and atomic weights of elements
Primarily legend	Generic and trade	U.S.	Current	Cost index for relative cost; tables for product comparison
Non-legend	Trade and generic	U.S.	Available in publication year	Monographs by different authors discuss types of preparation generally and give tabular data on individual preparations
Legend and non-legend	Trade and generic	Canadian	Current in 1967	Pictorial guide supplements basic codes and provides a limited index to them
Single entities	Trade, generic, chemical, and laboratory numbers	International	Current	Structural formulas provided. New items identified by black dot
Primarily legend	Generic (in Latin and English) and chemical	International	1953-1971	Includes procedures for selecting and devising international nonproprietary names
Primarily legend	Generic (in Latin and English) and chemical	International	Current in 1967	Includes structures and molecular formulas. 69 appendixes, mostly tests, but also lists of test reagents, reference substances, doses, weights, and measures. Lists of additions, deletions, alterations, and definitions at front
Single entities; investigational	Generic, trade, and chemical	General	General	Part 1 describes analytical techniques by type. Part 3 indexes from analytical data to compounds. Also includes reagent list and test index. Structures and chemical processes throughout
Primarily legend	Generic and trade	U.S.	Current	Special articles include effects of drugs on laboratory tests, summary of therapeutic measures for various kinds of cancer, etc. Occasional information on relative costs

Table 2. Editorial Aspects of Drug Handbooks

NAME	AUTHORITY	PURPOSE	GENERAL SCOPE
Merck Index	Commercial	To provide an index to organic chemicals, mostly of medicinal significance	10,000 organic chemicals plus a few natural mixtures and inorganic substances of medical importance
Modern Drug Encyclopedia & Modern Drugs	Commercial	To provide comprehensive and objective information on prescription drugs	Nationally distributed prescription drugs of 92 manufacturers
National Formulary	American Pharmaceutical Association; U.S. Pharmacopeial Convention beginning in 1975	To provide standards of identity, strength, quality, and purity for drugs of therapeutic value not in the *USP*	1,009 articles admitted in 14th revision in broad range of therapeutic categories
Negwer	Commercial	To provide basic information and worldwide synonyms for commonly used drugs	5,228 organic chemical medicinal substances with more than 40,000 synonyms
New Drugs	American Medical Association Council on Drugs	To provide "up-to-date, authoritative, and unbiased information on the more recently introduced drugs"	Monographs on drugs introduced during the 10 years before 1967 — date of last issue — and comparative reviews of older drugs, not necessarily endorsed or recommended by the AMA Council
Pharmacological and Chemical Synonyms	Commercial	To collect under a single heading all known names for a given substance	Approximately 9,000 headings and 25,000 synonyms from world medical literature
pharmIndex	Commercial	To provide comprehensive information on drug products and their packaging and price	Approximately 4,200 drug products distributed locally or nationally by about 275 companies
Physicians' Desk Reference and Supplements	Commercial	To present detailed and authoritative information provided by manufacturer and approved by Food and Drug Administration	About 250 companies list some 2,500 drug product monographs

Table 2. Editorial Aspects of Drug Handbooks

TYPE OF DRUG	COVERAGE BY: TYPE OF NAME	COUNTRY	TIME	SPECIAL FEATURES
Single entities	Chemical, generic, trade, and laboratory numbers	International	Current and established	Extensive appendixes including organic name reactions, first aid in poisoning, Greek and Russian alphabets, formula index to monographs. Most important is the cross index to names in the monograph section
Primarily legend	Generic and trade	U.S.	Currently marketed	List of trade names for dosage forms such as Tabloid and Spansule used with many different drugs. Special monographs for groups such as adrenal corticosteroids
Primarily legend, aids, and adjuncts	Generic and chemical	U.S.	Current	Much background on *National Formulary* operations and standards in introduction. Pharmaceutic aids and drugs in separate alphabets. Sections on general tests, etc., reagents and solutions, and tables, including a comparison between *NF* and *IP* standards and a list of former names of some *NF XIV* admissions
Single entities	Generic, chemical, trade, and laboratory numbers	All	Current and established	An interesting index by chemical rings and functional groups, such as aldehydes or indoles. Supplements to both the list and the index should not be overlooked
Primarily legend	Generic, trade, and chemical	U.S.	Current in 1967	Structural formulas and dates of introduction for drugs in monographs. Supplementary list of Canadian trade names for drugs in monographs. Discussion of official standards and regulatory agencies and *USAN* guidelines for nomenclature. Tables include children's dosage
Single entities, legend and non-legend	Generic, chemical, trade, and laboratory numbers	International	Current	Chemical names included in index
Primarily legend	Trade and generic; laboratory numbers in pending section	U.S.	Currently marketed	Separate review articles and products pending sections. Deleted products identified, and product and price changes listed
Primarily legend	Generic, trade, and common chemical	U.S.	Currently promoted by manufacturer	Drug codes listed for many manufacturers. Diagnostic section initiated in 1974; management of drug overdose, in 1975. Product identification section picturing over 1,000 tablets and capsules. Manufacturers' index includes phone numbers and inquiry and local addresses

Table 2. Editorial Aspects of Drug Handbooks

NAME	AUTHORITY	PURPOSE	GENERAL SCOPE
Red Book and Supplements, Drug Topics	Commercial	To provide a precise and complete source of information on availability, form, package, and prices of marketed drug products	All marketed products in general drug and sundries categories
USAN and the USP Dictionary of Drug Names	USAN Council sponsored by American Medical Association, U.S. Pharmacopeial Convention, and American Pharmaceutical Association, with liaison from Food and Drug Administration	To follow established principles to select a single, good nonproprietary name for "each promising new drug" and to cooperate in international acceptance of that name	Names adopted since June 15, 1961
U. S. Pharmacopeia	United States Pharmacopeial Convention, Inc.	To provide a select list of therapeutic substances together with standards of quality, strength, purity, and identity	1,300 drugs approved for admission as of high therapeutic utility
Unlisted Drugs and Index Guide	Commercial; initiated by Pharmacopeial Division, Special Libraries Association	To give brief information and reference sources for drugs not listed in specified common sources; *Index Guide* provides a cumulated index to the UD issues for the past 25 years	Some 2,000 new names and their identification each year, mostly newly marketed, foreign, or investigational drugs; about 80,000 entries in the cumulated Index Guide
Veterinarians' Blue Book	Commercial	To provide a source of information on veterinary drugs similar to the human drug handbooks	Includes foods, feed additives, and biologicals as well as drugs

Table 2. Editorial Aspects of Drug Handbooks

TYPE OF DRUG	COVERAGE BY:			SPECIAL FEATURES
	TYPE OF NAME	COUNTRY	TIME	
Legend and non-legend	Trade and sometimes generic	U.S.	Currently marketed	Product identification section for about 350 tablets, capsules and suppositories. Lists of drug interactions and numerous tables
Primarily legend	Generic, chemical, trade, and laboratory numbers	U.S.	Studied 1961-date	Separate listing of *USAN* and compendial names by therapeutic category; list of manufacturers of *USAN*; list of *USAN* by molecular formulas; CAS numbers
Primarily legend	Generic	U.S.	Current	Historical material and definitions plus sections on tests, processes and apparatus, and reagents, indicators, and solutions. Several tables. Separate sections for Drug Substances and Dosage Forms and Pharmaceutic Ingredients
Legend, non-legend, and investigational	Generic, chemical, trade, and laboratory numbers	All	Currently listed in literature; past 25 years for *Index Guide*	Each monthly issue contains reviews of new books and sometimes a summary of new drugs of interest. Graphic formulas are included. Also available on cards. Besides a world-wide manufacturers' address list, there is a separate section on manufacturers' codes associated with laboratory numbers in *Index Guide*
Combinations and single entities	Trade and generic	U.S.	Current in 1967	Special chapters and charts are inserted throughout the book. Examples are: breeding chart, average gestation period, recent books of significance, purpose of the F.D.A. etc. Note: For just over 200 drugs, Hansell, Dan N. and John D. Scheu, *Comparative Guide of Veterinary and Human Pharmaceuticals* (American Pharmaceutical Association, 2215 Constitution Ave., N.W., Washington, D.C. 20037, 1973, $4.00) supplements VBB with more current information.

coverage of drugs and chemicals that also describes adverse effects (in this case *Merck Index*), or one which tends to have very detailed monographs and gives references to the literature, so that one can pursue the question further. One such source, the *U.S. Dispensatory* — particularly in the 25th and previous editions — is also useful for older drugs and nonproprietaries, such as milk of magnesia, which often do not appear in either general handbooks or those on toxicology.

Physical incompatibilities. Many of the established drug handbooks have not yet adopted the term "drug interactions," although one will find information on such interactions under such terms as "incompatibilities." As implied by the terms, physical incompatibilities are those which occur between two drugs, or a drug and another chemical, outside the body, and therapeutic incompatibilities or interactions are those which occur when two drugs are used in the same person concurrently.

It is therapeutic incompatibilities which are generally meant when the term "drug interactions" is used today. If one wants extensive coverage, it would be wise also to use some of the various drug interactions handbooks and bibliographies which are appearing rapidly (See Chapter 8). In Table 1, handbooks which are checked for adverse reactions and are evaluative and frequently updated (e.g., *Medical Letter, AMA Drug Evaluations, American Hospital Formulary Service*) will be the best sources for drug interactions questions.

What is the dose of Farmlit for an adult? For a seven-year-old? How rapidly is it metabolized, i.e., how frequently can the dose be administered without a cumulative effect? and What is it used for? (Dosage; Pharmacology & Metabolism; Therapeutic Use)

Questions as simple as one involving the usual dose of a particular product can be answered in any of the sources checked in the dosage column in Table 1, whether or not they contain information on pharmacology and metabolism as well. If you want to know whether to alter dosage for people with renal insufficiency, or if you need specifications of doses for children, you are more likely to find such information in books that deal with metabolism and pharmacology as well as dosage. A single column was used for metabolism and pharmacology because most books that include one also have some information on the other.

Similarly, all sources marked with a plus in the Therapeutic Use column will name the "indication" for the drug. Information on how or why you use it to treat the disease will probably be found in those texts which include information on pharmacology and metabolism as well as on therapeutic use.

How can I tell whether an overdose of Farmlit was the cause of death in this suicide? There were some tablets in the patient's purse which are not labeled; how can I tell what they might be by looking at them? (Physical and Chemical Properties; Physical Identification)

In modern-day pharmacy, we may not often need to know the solubility or specific gravity of a tablet, and relatively few of the sources listed contain this sort of information. The British *Isolation and Identification of Drugs* is directed specifically to the need to identify poisonous substances, particularly in biological materials.

Not infrequently a physician or patient, tablet or capsule in hand, will want to know what it is. While positive identification can be made only by physical analysis, it may not be possible to wait. One can still count on the fingers of one hand the places where he can turn for help, and none are complete. Each of the sources marked in the Physical Identification column has pictures of some of the tablets and capsules one may encounter, and identifies the drug. *Identification Guide*, by Gupta and Kofoed, gives many more details on size, shape, and scoring, for more drugs. But this careful and detailed analysis makes the book more difficult to use, and the demand for the book is apparently not sufficient to allow keeping it up to date. In addition, since it is published in Canada, many American products are missing, even though it is the most extensive listing presently available.

When was Farmlit discovered, patented, first marketed? (History of Drug)

In the pharmaceutical industry, such questions may be asked because they relate to the possibility of marketing the drug. The user of the drug probably does not very often care how it got into the armamentarium, but the person seeking information in the literature will find that knowing the history of the drug helps him search for information on it. Most of the papers on its pharmacology in animals are likely to have been published within two to five years of the initial chemical paper. Certainly, there are not likely to be articles on clinical use of a drug much before the first chemical paper. They do occur because of the vagaries of publishing, but in a relatively short time span.

Where can I find more about Farmlit? (References to Other Sources)

As can be seen in Table 1, relatively few of the handbooks provide references to journal articles or other sources of additional information. When they do, the papers are apt to be selected and are thus among the most important available at the time of publication. An exception is *Unlisted Drugs,* where the reference given is the *first* noted by the publishers, not necessarily the best or even very informative.

CHAPTER **4**

LOOKING AT THE HANDBOOK

While the kind of question to be answered can get one into the right ballpark (or group of handbooks), it takes a more detailed knowledge of the individual handbook to know which to consult first for a given question. The preferred source can depend upon the questioner (is it a physician, a research worker, a nurse?), upon the urgency of the need for an answer (is it needed for treatment of an acutely ill patient within the next few minutes?), and upon the drug involved (does it appear to be used in the United States frequently, rarely, or not at all? is a prescription required for its use?). No two books provide exactly the same information, even though a few (such as *Red Book* and *Blue Book*) are closely competitive. The book that you will turn to first in a given situation will depend upon its purpose or the audience to which it is directed; its authority, scope, and coverage in terms of numbers of drugs as well as kinds of drug and kinds of name; and its geographic and chronologic extent. Occasionally a specific feature, such as a special table, will be needed. All these elements of the handbooks are discussed below and in Table 2. Other things being equal, one may decide which source to use on the basis of its format, or of the frequency with which it is updated and how conveniently it is cumulated. These elements are compared in Table 3.

Table 3. Format Aspects of Drug Handbooks

SHORT NAME	MAJOR ACCESS POINT(S)	ARRANGEMENT	INDEXES BY: GENERIC NAME*	TRADE NAME*	INDICA-TION*
ADT	Therapeutic class in Section II (Therapeutic Agents)	Classified	G	G	G
AMA-DE	Therapeutic class	Classified	C	C	—
ADI	Any name in dictionary style, including some action groups	Alphabetic	T	T	T
AHFS	Therapeutic class, subdivided by alphabetic generic names	Classified	G	G	G
Blue Book	Drug product trade name	Alphabetic	T	T	—
CPS	Trade name, or occasionally generic	Alphabetic	T,L	T,L	L
Current Drug Handbook	Therapeutic class	Classified	G	G	G
de Haen NNI	Various kinds as indicated by indexes	Alphabetic	L	L	L
Dispensatory (U.S.)	Generic or common name, plus a few drug classes	Alphabetic	T,C	C	L
Drugs of Choice	Therapeutic action	Classified	G,L	G,L	G
Drugs in Current Use	Generic name	Alphabetic in two sections	T	T	—
EP	Name of prototype or activity for each compound group	Alphabetic	C	C	S
Facts and Comparisons	Therapeutic groups	Classified	G	G	G
HND	Monographs on groups of drugs and sundries	Classified	—	S	—
Identification Guide	Form, e.g., tablets or capsules, and code number based on characteristics	Numerical	—	—	—
Index Nominum	French form of international nonproprietary name	Alphabetic	T	T	—
INN	Latin form of international nonproprietary name	Alphabetic	T	—	—
International Pharmacopoeia	Latin form of international nonproprietary name	Alphabetic	T,G	—	—

DRUG HANDBOOKS 21

Table 3. Format Aspects of Drug Handbooks

MANUFAC-TURER*	OTHER INDEXES	PHYSICAL FORM*	PERIODICITY	MOST RECENT PUBLICATION DATE IF NOT ANNUAL
L		Bound Volume	Biennial	1973/1974, 35th ed.
L	Adverse reactions	Bound Volume	Irregular	1973, 2nd ed.
L		Bound Volume	Annual	
—		U	Continuing supplements for insertion in basic volume	
L		Bound Volume	Annual	
L		Bound Volume	Annual, updated by "New Pharmaceuticals" section of *Canadian Pharmaceutical Journal* and *Canadian Medical Association Journal*	
—		Bound Volume	Biennial	1974/1976
S	European & Japanese products	Bound Volume	Irregular	1974, vol. 9
—		Bound Volume	Irregular	1973, 27th ed.
—		Bound Volume	Biennial	1974/1975
—		Bound Volume	Annual	
L		Bound Volume	Irregular	1972, 26th ed.
—		U	Monthly supplements for insertion in basic volume	
S		Bound Volume	Biennial	1973, 3rd ed.
—		U	Planned supplements have not been issued. Another edition unlikely	1967
—		Bound Volume	Biennial	1975/1976
—	Molecular formula	Bound Volume	Updated by frequent supplements in *WHO Chronicle*	1971, Cumulative List No. 3
—		Bound Volume	Irregular; occasional supplements	1967, 2nd ed. 1971 supplement

*See footnote for Table 3, page 24

Table 3. Format Aspects of Drug Handbooks (continued)

SHORT NAME	MAJOR ACCESS POINT(S)	ARRANGEMENT	INDEXES BY: GENERIC NAME*	TRADE NAME*	INDICATION*
Isolation and Identification of Drugs	(1) Type of procedure or test; (2) generic name	(1) Classified; (2) Alphabetic	T,G	G	G
Medical Letter	Generic name	Not applicable. Only 1 or 2 monographs per issue	G	G	G
Merck Index	Generic or common chemical name	Alphabetic	T,C	C	—
Modern Drug Encyclopedia	Trade or generic name	Alphabetic	T,C	T,C	S
NF	Generic name	Alphabetic in two sections	T,G	—	G,L
Negwer	Generic or Trade name; drugs arranged by incremental molecular formulas, C's and H's first, then other atoms in alphabetical order	Alphanumeric by ascending number of C's, etc.	C	C	—
New Drugs	Therapeutic class	Classified	G	G	G
Pharmacological and Chemical Synonyms	Any name, in dictionary style	Alphabetic	T	T	—
pharmIndex	Trade Name	Alphabetic	S	T,S	S
PDR	Company, with product subdivision	Alphabetic	S	S	S
Red Book	Trade name; occasionally generic	Alphabetic	T	T	—
USAN/USP-DDN	Generic name, brand name, code designation	Alphabetic	T	T	S
USP	Generic name	Alphabetic in two sections	T,G	—	G,L
UD	Separate sections for any name and for laboratory numbers	Alphabetic and numeric, respectively	T,C	T,C	—
Veterinarians' Blue Book	Broad groups such as Drugs and Biologicals, Small Animal Foods, and Feed Additives	Alphabetic	T	T	S

Table 3. Format Aspects of Drug Handbooks (continued)

MANUFAC-TURER*	OTHER INDEXES	PHYSICAL FORM*	PERIODICITY	MOST RECENT PUBLICATION DATE IF NOT ANNUAL
—		Bound Volumes	Irregular	Vol. 1, 1969; Vol. 2, 1975
—		U	Fortnightly, with quarterly cumulating indexes, up to annual, and also cumulative indexes to vols. 1-6 and 7-12	
—		Bound Volume	Irregular	1968, 8th ed.
S		Bound Volume	Irregular. *Modern Drugs* published periodically as a supplement	1975, 13th ed.
—		Bound Volume	Every 5 years, with several supplements between bound volumes	1975, 14th rev.
—	Group index of chemicals	Bound Volume	Irregular. 4th ed. in 2 volumes	1971, 4th ed.
L		Bound Volume	Annual for 3 years, preceded by *New and Nonofficial Drugs* and followed by *AMA Drug Evaluations*, which see	1967
—		Bound Volume	Irregular	1973, 5th ed.
S	Products pending and reviews	U	Monthly with cumulation of indexes to annual	
T,S		Bound Volume	Annual with 2 supplements at 4-month intervals	
L		Bound Volume	Annual, with 2 supplements at 4-month intervals	
L	Molecular formula and CAS numbers	Bound Volume	Annual	
—		Bound Volume	Every 5 years, with several supplements between bound volumes	1975, 19th rev.
L (*Index Guide*)	Manufacturer code letter keys in *Index Guide*	U or cards	Monthly, with semiannual, annual and biennial indexes. Earlier cumulations superseded by *Index Guide,* 1949-1967, *Index Guide II,* 1949-1970, *Index Guide III,* 1949-1973	
S		Bound Volume	Publication, which had been annual was temporarily suspended	1967, 15th ed.

*See footnote for Table 3, next page

FOOTNOTES FOR TABLE 3

*Abbreviations: C = Combination of generic and trade names in a single index
  G = General index includes item indicated
  L = Listed separately without reference to other parts of volume
  S = Separate index
  T = Text (body of book includes this item alphabetically)
  U = Updated by looseleaf additions

Authority

Historically, there have been a number of groups that pass on drugs, creating standards for purity, efficacy, nomenclature, etc. Sometimes it is difficult to tell exactly what such sources are standardizing. They may provide an authoritative name for a drug and give descriptive data incidentally, or their primary interest may be in the standards of purity or efficacy, and only secondarily in the names. Standards for names as such will be discussed under *Kind of Name*.

In the United States, drugs were regulated by physicians and pharmacists long before the federal government was involved. In 1820 a group of physicians representing medical societies and schools in the various districts of the United States assembled in Washington, D.C. as the first United States Pharmacopeial Convention. They organized, adopting a constitution and bylaws, and reviewed and consolidated draft pharmacopeias, which became the first *U.S. Pharmacopeia* on December 15, 1820. It contained 217 drugs considered worthy of recognition. Thereafter, the conventions have met every ten years. Until 1940, the *Pharmacopeia* was revised every ten years; thereafter, every five years. Although the first convention was composed exclusively of physicians, in the second and third conventions prominent pharmacists assisted, and in 1850 pharmacists were given full membership. The *Pharmacopeia* has represented the most authoritative source of standards for drugs for over a century, both in the United States and in many other countries, particularly in Latin America, where it has been translated into Spanish and frequently adopted as official.

However, a number of other authoritative bodies have been organized to supplement the work of the *Pharmacopeia* in a variety of ways. Since the *U.S. Pharmacopeia (USP)* was limited to drugs selected as having "the greatest therapeutic merit," pharmacists were early aware of a great many drugs with a substantial degree of acceptance for which standards were not available in the *USP*. Consequently, the American Pharmaceutical Association, in 1888, published the first edition of the *National Formulary of Unofficial Preparations (NF)*.

Thus, in 1906, when the first Federal Food and Drugs Act was passed, there were two reliable sources of standards available. Rather than start from scratch, the Act recognized the standards of the *USP* and *NF* as those with which drugs described therein must comply. Thus, at the same time, the publications and their standards were given legal status, and the self-regulation implied in sponsorship of the two publications by representative professional bodies was maintained.

Because of the need for close coordination between the two publications, the *National Formulary* was acquired by the USP Convention, Inc., immediately following publication of *National Formulary XIV* and future revisions will be published by the USP group.

There are two other professional groups that have created and published handbooks of standards in the field. The American Medical Association recognized a gap between the drugs and drug products admitted to the *USP* and *NF* and the new remedies which were appearing. Progressive physicians wanted unbiased information on such remedies from their peers. So another "nonofficial" source was created, *New and Nonofficial Remedies (NNR)*, which reached the status of a standard-maker as manufacturers filed new drug information with the AMA Council on Drugs at the same time they submitted it to the Food and Drug Administration.

Certain rules were established for admission of materials to *NNR*, including among others the requirements that their composition be disclosed and suitable tests for identity and purity be provided to the Council on Pharmacy and Chemistry. In addition, the drugs included were not to be advertised to the general public. The AMA was able to get such cooperation from the producer of drugs because it was desirable to have the drug listed in its *NNR*, and acceptance in that publication was for many years a condition of using the AMA Seal of Acceptance on packages and advertising for the drug. In 1955, the AMA dropped the Seal of Acceptance and in 1958, it changed the publication's name to *New and Nonofficial Drugs*. In 1964, the publication in that format was discontinued.

When the Food and Drug Administration began legally to pass on the efficacy as well as safety of every new drug before it was allowed to be sold in interstate commerce, the term "nonofficial" lost its former meaning. All approved new drugs have legal status, whether or not they are "official" in *USP* or *NF*. But the need for unbiased, nonlegal information on drugs remains, and perhaps is more urgent, as drugs become more potent and knowledge about them more esoteric.

At the same time, after its introduction in the late 1940's, the *Physician's Desk Reference (PDR)*, had become the physician's "bible" because it was distributed free of charge to every physician, resident and intern in the United States, and even to students in medicine and the other health professions. The economics were simple. The drug manufacturer paid *Physician's Desk Reference* for every entry on its drugs which appeared in *PDR*. Because he paid, he chose which drugs would appear in *PDR* and supplied the copy. Often physicians were unaware that they were subject to the bias of the manufacturer just as much as if they listened to his detailman or read his "junk mail."

Partly to combat the ubiquity of the *PDR*, and partly for the purposes which had established the predecessor *NNR* and *NND*, the AMA attempted to produce an inexpensive, easy-to-use, authoritative and unbiased drug handbook in *New Drugs*, which appeared in 1965, 1966, and 1967. While *New Drugs* was subtitled "Evaluated by the AMA," and did include many clinical judgments, it was difficult to weigh and review opinions and produce a truly evaluative text on an annual basis. Since such a text was sorely needed and uniquely within its province, the AMA Council on Drugs labored long and critically and brought forth the *AMA Drug Evaluations*, first edition, in 1971. A second edition appeared in 1973. Like their predecessor, they include more detail about drugs that have been introduced in the previous ten years and those in the official compendia. They list essentially all single entities dispensed exclusively or principally by prescription as well as the mixtures most commonly prescribed. Many of the monographs used in the 1967 *New Drugs* were revised only slightly in the 1971 edition, but the revisions were generally in the direction of more positive and critical statements.

Meanwhile, hospital pharmacists were faced with similar, but different problems. They were concerned, of course, that the physician in the hospital have adequate and unbiased guidance in his choice of drugs. But in addition, it was necessary for the hospital pharmacy to control costs, through some rationalization of the drugs which would be stocked. Many hospitals have formularies, which list the drugs that may be prescribed routinely by their staff. To make it easier for them to prepare such formularies, and to provide a standard which they could adopt wholly or partially, the first American Hospital Formulary Service was produced in 1959. This is perhaps the most useful to the hospital pharmacists of all the tools mentioned, since it is prepared by and for them.

Gradually, as legislation has given the Food and Drug Administration additional authority, it has come out with publications of its own intended to supersede other authorities in any respect in which they differ. However, they have relied heavily on the existing "official" sources, *USP* and *NF*, and thus have not been in conflict.

In general, publications of the FDA are of minor interest to the pharmacist, because the results of the regulations reach him through other channels. The official statements appear in Title 21 of the *Code of Federal Regulations*, which gives all the rules promulgated by the FDA. It is supplemented by announcements in the *Federal Register*. Here can be found up-to-date lists of names approved by the FDA which are cumulated also in each edition of *USAN*.

While the package insert has for many years been a combination of informational and promotional literature, it now has legal status because the FDA requires that those drugs having "official" package circulars must use approved labeling language verbatim for such information as action, dose, and hazards. Through a strange quirk of fate, the *Physician's Desk Reference*, which was criticized in the past because of its sponsorship by manufacturers, now includes essentially the package inserts as its monographs and is thus a source of official descriptions of a drug's actions, contraindications, dosage, etc., as approved by the FDA. It is now sometimes criticized because it includes a mass of undigested information. A caution against an adverse reaction does not indicate whether it has occurred once in 100 or once in 100,000 administrations of the drug. Many minor drugs are not included in *PDR* because the manufacturer does not choose to pay to list them.

Each country has its own series of authoritative handbooks, the number and variety depending on the history of pharmacy and political organization in the country. The Pharmaceutical Society of Great Britain, for instance, publishes the *British Pharmacopoeia*, the *British National Formulary*, and the *British Pharmaceutical Codex*, as well as the *Extra Pharmacopoeia* and *British Veterinary Codex*, thus in effect being responsible for all the official British publications.

Except for a few with international coverage, foreign sources are not listed here, but the reader should know they are available and how to find them. Several detailed lists can be found. (See, for example, Bloomfield, Pasztor and Hopkins, and the Special Libraries Association's *Drug Information Sources* in Table 5.) Many libraries do not have complete sets of such handbooks, both because of the lack of questions about foreign drugs, and because of the effort to keep them up to date. Many are published by pharmaceutical associations or other nontrade publishers, and are not announced in the regular library sources. If a pharmacist is in an area where there is a large community of recent immigrants or there are regular foreign visitors, he may wish to cooperate in the acquisition of suitable sources for identification of foreign drugs.

Purposes of Handbooks

In the preceding section, the purposes of the authoritative handbooks were defined in discussing why their sponsors published them. That these did not satisfy all of the needs for information is evident from the number of commercial publishers of drug handbooks. Each found a gap in available publications which it believed it could fill, hopefully with financial benefit.

Merck Index is "an encyclopedia of chemicals and drugs," and as such, the most extensive of all drug handbooks. *American Drug Index* and *Pharmacological and Chemical Synonyms* are dictionaries giving minimal, but useful information on many drugs in a single, alphabetical list. They provide a ready resource when one is not sure if a name is an official name, a trade name, or purely a chemical description.

Modern Drug Encyclopedia is the ancestor of all comprehensive commercial handbooks limited to drugs. (*Merck Index* appeared earlier.) It was produced first in 1935 and is now in its 13th edition. A similar compendium is *pharmIndex*, except that its updating mechanism is integral to the publication, since it is looseleaf, whereas *MDE* is updated by a periodical supplement, *Modern Drugs*. Because it is extensive with respect to the drugs it includes, and also gives packaging and price information, *pharmIndex* tends to be used more by pharmacists than by physicians. It has extra features, including a section on investigational drugs, which are found rarely elsewhere.

Community pharmacists are familiar with the *American Druggist Blue Book* and *Drug Topics Red Book*, and know them as sources of information for price, size, dosage form, and manufacturer. But are they aware of the comparison of costs to be found in *Facts and Comparisons*?

Several commercial publishers issue evaluative information. Noteworthy among them are *Medical Letter* and Modell's *Drugs of Choice*.

Each profession has one or more drug compendia of its own, examples being *Accepted Dental Therapeutics* for dentists, *Current Drug Handbook* for nurses, and *Veterinarian's Blue Book* for veterinarians.

Even the pharmacist who has little call to identify foreign drugs may wish to have one of the sources which list foreign drugs generally regardless of their country of origin. Perhaps most useful, because of the other information it includes, is *Extra Pharmacopoeia*. However, it is reissued only about every five years, and can be out of date when current information is needed. The same is true of Negwer's *Organisch-chemische Arzneimittel und ihre Synonyma*, which has more extensive coverage of drugs and synonyms. The nonGerman speaking reader should not be turned away by the title, because the synonyms given are in all languages and it requires little ingenuity to translate Kamaver to chloramphenicol when they are both on the synonym list for the same chemical substance. The chemical structures and molecular formulas are also not language-dependent. In the fourth edition, the preface and introduction are translated into English.

Finally, *Unlisted Drugs (UD)*, though not initiated by a commercial organization, is presently published by one. A group of librarians in the Pharmaceutical Division of the Special Libraries

Association noted a need for a means of identifying investigational drugs and others not yet on the market as well as new foreign drugs not in standard lists. In January 1949, *Unlisted Drugs* was born as a cooperative publication of this group. Its recent cumulative indexes, *Index Guides*, 1949-1967, 1949-1970 and 1949-1973, cover cumulatively more entries than any of the other sources, although one must have access to a complete set of the monthly *UD* in order to find the data referred to. It should be noted that essentially all the information in *UD* comes from secondary sources — mostly advertisements, notices, or original articles in journals — and little effort was made to update it if later publications brought out new information, at least during the thirteen years when it was being edited (as a labor of love!) by the author of this *Guide to Drug Information*.

Scope and Coverage

The purpose for which a handbook is intended and its general scope and coverage are usually interwoven. If the scope of the source is broad, it is quite likely, however, to be used for purposes for which it was not originally devised. *Unlisted Drugs*, for instance, lists so many laboratory numbers that it was a good source for linking alphabetic codes with manufacturer even before the list of codes was published in its *Index Guide*. A group of students doing an assignment on general properties and uses of drugs found Clarke's *Isolation and Identification of Drugs* close to the more general handbooks on the library shelves and used it along with *Extra Pharmacopoeia*. Perhaps they couldn't find anything in Clarke that they couldn't also get from the more general source, but they managed to locate all they needed.

Some aspects of coverage by drug handbooks, for example geographic and chronological, require little discussion. On the other hand, selectivity of coverage — while often desirable — will determine the number of drugs in the list and thus the likelihood of finding Farmlit — or whatever the drug of immediate interest. Besides being aware of the quantity of drugs listed, it is important to understand as clearly as possible the kind of drug or chemical substance included, and the kinds of name one may encounter. These two items are discussed separately.

Kind of Drug

The best source in the world is no good to us at the moment

if it doesn't contain information on the particular drug or drug name we are looking for. Probably the major reason there are so many sources is that there are so many different drugs available in so many different parts of the world under so many different names. When we realize that the U.S. *Pharmacopeia* and the *National Formulary* each cover only about 1,000 drugs, the problem seems relatively simple. Even the sources which cover most of the "ethical" or "prescription" drugs in the United States include well under 5,000. The *Physician's Desk Reference*, for example, appears — from a check of the generic name index — to include about 1,000 different entities, although the introduction says it contains over 2,500 products. *pharmIndex*, with its inclusion of many drugs distributed locally, appears to list about 1,600 different substances, with 8,600 different trade names.

How does one characterize drugs in order to distinguish between the kind contained in one book and that which appears in another? In the *Handbook of Non-Prescription Drugs*, Griffenhagen and Hawkins speak of the "jargon jungle" of terminology with relation to self-medication products.[1] (Self-medication itself appears in the Canadian and British literature as automedication.)

The problem with making such distinctions is that a number of lines are drawn, none of them very clearly: Smith and Knapp[2] make a useful and precise division between "legend" and "nonlegend" drugs. They define "legend" drugs as those to which the following legend (or statement) applies: *"Caution: Federal Law Prohibits Dispensing Without a Prescription."* They point out that not all prescribed drugs are legend drugs, but that legend drugs must be prescribed before they may be dispensed. While this is a useful distinction in describing the kinds of materials contained in handbooks, the books are not usually divided purely along these lines. At the core of the physician's armamentarium, such substances as aspirin are usually included in lists primarily limited to legend drugs. And so the line between legend and nonlegend, or "over-the-counter" drugs, is somewhat indistinct.

One soon observes that there is a fairly clear differentiation between single entities and combinations. The single entities are largely patented prescription products marketed by a single manufacturer under a single trade name, and the combinations are mostly nostrums containing several well-known and relatively harmless ingredients marketed by individual companies under a given trade name, but whose equivalents may be found under different names and slightly different formulas distributed by hundreds of other companies. The distinction is almost the same as that between legend and nonlegend, but the line is not clear because some single entities are not legend-only drugs, and some combinations are. (The oral contraceptives are the most modern example of the latter.)

One interesting possibility for distinction among the various sources is to separate those which list drugs from those which enumerate drug products. By "drug," we mean the active ingredient of a preparation, the component measured in calculating the usual dosage in relation to the anticipated activity. By "drug product," we mean that tablet or capsule or ampule which is presented to the patient, complete with its inert ingredients. Naturally a publication which lists drug products contains many more entries than one which lists drugs only. Even if the latter provides trade names, it is still naming a class of drug products, because the same trade name may be used with a number of different forms of the drug. In our experience, those sources which list drug products tend to have broader scope in terms of listing both legend and nonlegend drugs. But this does not hold true for the dictionaries, particularly *American Drug Index*, which contains essentially no information on product form, but which is full of guides to trade names for combinations, many of which are nonlegend drugs.

Thus guidance is needed, but no clear-cut distinction is available. We have followed the scope and coverage guidelines of the particular sources with which we are dealing. If the criterion for inclusion is therapeutic value, as with the *USP* and *NF*, then we have indicated in Table 2 that the kind of drug included is primarily legend, even though some of the specific drugs may be available without a prescription as well. If all drug products are included, as with the *Red Book* and *Blue Book*, we have said that the kind of drug included is legend and nonlegend. If single entities are the major guideline, as with *Merck* and *Negwer*, we have so indicated, hoping the user will infer that the compounds therein cross boundaries between legend, nonlegend, and investigational drugs.

At best, this kind of distinction in relation to handbooks can serve as a sort of negative guide. One would not look in *Modern Drug Encyclopedia*, *PDR*, or the *Red Book* or *Blue Book* for investigational drugs unless one had some reason to believe they might already be marketed. If one were looking for the composition of a nonlegend drug, he would start with *American Drug Index* or the *Handbook of Non-Prescription Drugs* (depending on his need for the precise formulation); he would not turn to USP.

It is usually more difficult to find information about drugs not on the market (either investigational or deleted) than those marketed. For this reason, Table 2 identifies sources which cover them.

Kind of Name

Ten years ago, we were quoting Dr. Miller, then Director of Revision of the *U.S. Pharmacopeia*: "What perplexes students and practicing physicians alike is why these drugs must be known by seldom fewer than three, usually four, and often more than a half-dozen different names. And those who go abroad for study find themselves obliged to learn still other names in use there for familiar drugs."[3] The situation is not entirely changed today, but we are moving toward greater simplicity.

There is an organization for naming a drug, which is not concerned with evaluating the product itself. If there is a chance that a chemical may be considered for marketing, the manufacturer may submit a nonproprietary name to the United States Adopted Names Council. This name is called nonproprietary because by definition it is not subject to proprietary or trademark rights. It is frequently also referred to as generic, although the latter is a more ambiguous term. In a sense, the nonproprietary name protects the trademark of the manufacturer, because only the manufacturer's product may be referred to by the trademark, and any other reference to the product must use the nonproprietary name. Before nonproprietary names were so routinely and carefully applied to each product, a proprietary name could be declared "in the common domain" because of its frequent uncontested use when the company product was not specifically referred to. "Adrenalin" started out as a trademark, but — spelled with an "e" — it is a nonproprietary name in the *British Pharmacopoeia*, and it is frequently referred to in that way in this country as well, even though the *USP* nonproprietary name is "epinephrine."

The *USAN* Council is made up of three agencies: the American Medical Association, the U.S. Pharmacopeial Convention, and the American Pharmaceutical Association. They work through it with the FDA and with foreign nomenclature boards toward the goal that the name they adopt will be the worldwide name for the drug. There are still occasional and annoying spelling differences between *U.S. Adopted Names* and *International Nonproprietary Names.* The occasional differences are difficult to justify, since one of the reasons the new system works as well as it does is a rather cavalier disregard for orthography on the part of the naming boards. What chemist, for instance, likes to see the syllables "dione" limited to "antiepileptics derived from oxazolidinedione," or "medro," "meto," and "clo" being preferred to the more conventional substituent designations of "methylhydro," "methoxy," and "chlor," respectively? In any event, when there are minor spelling differences, they are not likely to block communication.

Names approved by the *USAN* Council may be considered to be official in the sense that the FDA has designated the *USP* and the *NF* names as official when it has not itself announced an official name. To date, the FDA has provided lists of some 500 official names which are published periodically in the *Federal Register* and are updated each year in the cumulation of *United States Adopted Names (USAN).*

There are other nonproprietary names which have no official status. Many of these are simply traditional names for a product. "Epsom salt" is a common name which is a synonym for the *USP* Magnesium Sulfate.

A drug may have more than one trade name, even in the same country, for different formulations. Nitrofurantoin, for instance, may be purchased as Macrodantin® and Furadantin® in different preparations from the same company, and other names are used by other companies in the United States and abroad. Products not protected by patents are apt to have a multiplicity of trade names. There are about fifty listed under penicillin G in *Pharmacological and Chemical Synonyms,* although the so-called synonyms are for both the potassium and sodium salts. If one is interested in the owner of a trade mark, he may consult *Trademarks Listed with the Pharmaceutical Manufacturers Association* (November 1970), a cumulative index to the *Bulletin of the Trademark Bureau of the PMA.* This index also contains coined nonproprietary names which have not been adopted by the USAN Council.

The trade name is probably the better known, but most of the sources marked in Table 1 for "Equivalent Identification" will translate both from nonproprietary to trade name and from trade to nonproprietary, so that identification in the United States is not difficult. For foreign identification, one would look to the few sources marked for all countries or as international in Table 2, or turn to the lists of foreign drug compendia cited in Table 5.

Something needs to be said of two other kinds of name, the chemical name and the code number. These will be a problem only if one deals with drugs in research in one way or another, but they can be considerable problems. In the first place, there can be almost as many different chemical names for a drug as there are chemists to name it; all can be accurate in the sense that one could draw a structural formula on the basis of one name and it would represent exactly the same chemical as the structural formulas drawn for each of the other names. But it is virtually impossible to list each chemical under all of its possible chemical names in a printed index. Therefore, nomenclature rules have been established. Most people who have taken an undergraduate chemistry course have heard of the International Union of Pure and Applied Chemistry (IUPAC) nomenclature rules. It is the extension of these rules and their application in the indexes of *Chemical Abstracts,* however, which is most important for use of the indexes to the handbooks we are discussing. *USAN* and *Merck Index,* for instance, give the preferred *Chemical Abstracts* name as the first synonym for the generic or common name. Though the chemical name is not an index or "entry" point in *USAN*, it is in *Merck Index,* and there one can find many chemical synonyms other than that preferred by *CA*. The point is that, if one knows the *CA* name, one can establish easily and definitely whether or not a particular drug or chemical is in the *Merck Index*. The best chance to find the chemical in the other sources, too, is to use the *CA* name. Occasionally there will be another chemical name that one has heard frequently which is likely to be used in the index. If all else fails, and one knows the structural formula, one can calculate the molecular formula and check it in *Negwer* or *Merck*.

We turn finally to the code name, or investigational, experimental, or laboratory number. Probably every pharmaceutical research laboratory in any part of the world has some systematic way of identifying the compounds its chemists have synthesized. Usually, it is a serial numbering system of some sort. When a compound is first reported in the literature — perhaps along with many other compounds in an article reporting on their screening for a particular purpose — it will be identified by a number plus some sort of identifier for the laboratory. Many of the prefixes are simply an abbreviation of the company name (BW for Burroughs Wellcome, Win for Winthrop Laboratories, SKF for Smith Kline and French, or Ro for Roche Laboratories). In other instances, they serve to identify different laboratories within a corporation (CIBA's Ba for its Basle laboratories and Su for those in Summit). In many other instances, it is impossible to guess from the letters which company made the product and, indeed, the letters are not always unique. In the list in *Unlisted Drugs Index Guide, 1949-1970* for instance, there are seventeen companies using the code letter "A," fifteen using "R" and even four using "LA."

The first place to look for individual investigational numbers is *UD* because it lists more of them. In addition, it lists them by number, so that one can ignore the puzzling variants of the same code designation which one encounters in other handbooks. For instance, L20025 is a Lilly drug, but in *Negwer* it is separated by two pages from the numbers preceded by Lilly in that alphabetical index. The same sort of situation can occur in any other index which lists code numbers alphabetically under their letters. Unfortunately, as with names, no single source is complete, so that all should be checked under all variants.

Finally, for the benefit of those who do not read foreign languages, I might add that the code letter in some foreign countries is usually placed after the number, just as an adjective is placed after a noun in the same languages. Don't let this disturb you. The compound is the same, either way.

Special Features

Occasionally a handbook may be kept for some special table it contains long after its basic information is out of date, yet these tables are frequently overlooked by those who have small collections and might have most use for them. It is impossible to list all the special features in such sources as *Merck Index*, the

Red Book, and the *Blue Book*, but I would encourage you to look at each new edition and to make a mental note of the useful items it contains. Fifteen minutes in advance may save you countless hours later.

Format Aspects

Most of the elements in Table 3 can as easily be observed by going directly to the sources, but it will be helpful to scan it to see what pitfalls one encounters. For instance, if you had occasion to use *International Nonproprietary Names*, which does not have an index, you might assume that clofenamic acid was not there because you didn't find it under "C." Wrong! It is there, but under the Latin name "acidum clofenamicum," and so on for all the acids!

We have already mentioned the fact that one cannot use *Merck Index* effectively without using the synonym index at the back. But look at all the possible permutations of indexes in Table 3, and beware of simply turning to the first index you see and assuming that if you don't find Farmlit, it isn't there! Also note the few unusual indexes which you may find particularly useful.

---

1. Griffenhagen, George B., and Hawkins, Linda L. "Introduction." In *Handbook of Non-Prescription Drugs, 1971 Edition*. American Pharmaceutical Association, Washington, D.C., 1971. p. 4.

2. Smith, Mickey C. and Knapp, David A. *Pharmacy, Drugs and Medical Care*. Williams & Wilkins Co., Baltimore, 1972. p. 154.

3. Miller, Lloyd C. "Doctors, Drugs, and Names." *Journal of the American Medical Association* 177:97, July 8, 1961.

CHAPTER 5

CHOOSING A PERSONAL COLLECTION

To this point, our primary approach has been to suggest what sources to use when answering a question or solving a problem. By implication, of course, that tells you which of them you may want to own. Since Table 5 contains a number of guides to book selection, we shall not try to include another book list here. We have starred in Table 1 the fourteen handbooks that probably should be in a minimal collection. In addition to sources listed in Table 5, a great many texts and handbooks have their own book lists, for example the *Red Book* and the *Blue Book*. In the latter, the list included in the section on a Medical Profile System in the 1971 edition is a good selection.

The final choice will have to be based on the needs and purposes of the individual, but I hope the tables on handbooks will be helpful. Probably you will want to determine the purpose, scope, and coverage of the information that is necessary in your work first, and to check Table 2 for the best sources to answer the need. After that, you might make sure that the sources are checked in Table 1 for answering the kinds of questions you would anticipate.

When the field has been narrowed on the basis of content, you will want to use Table 3 to consider convenience of use. There are aspects of format, such as adequate type size, pleasing appearance of information on the page, durable binding, and many others, which can be determined only by examining the book. We would recommend that you do so before making your final choice. However, a brief discussion of various methods of keeping the service up to date may be helpful. For each kind of very current service, there are costs in time as well as money, which must be compared to the rewards.

Annuals

These are usually quite current and easy to handle. Because of time lag in publication, one year's edition is probably a year and a half out of date by the time the next one is received. The more comprehensive and varied the information it includes, the more likely there are to be mistakes in an annual compilation. As an example, it is possible to find a number of mistakes in *American Drug Index*, in many ways the most generally useful of the annual compilations. For instance, Velban® is listed as an antineoplastic agent under the V's, but is not listed in the A's with other antineoplastic agents in the 1971 edition. In the same edition, Russel Viper Venom appears as a name without either definition or cross reference to tell one what it is all about!

Supplements to Annuals

These help to take care of the interval between annual issues, but, unless they are cumulated with each issue, tend to make more places to look the more frequent the issues. They also tend to get lost or forgotten when one is using the main volume.

Looseleaf Services

These may have the best cost-to-benefit ratio. With five minutes of effort when the supplementary material is received, one can maintain a current reference service which is relatively easy to use, with a minimum of places to look. Beware the chaos in your looseleaf volume, though, if you don't keep it properly filed! This happens all too frequently in libraries. If others do your filing, be sure of their intelligence and motivation!

Card Services

While no card services are included on the tables, there are a number available. The best known for the kind of information found in handbooks are mostly foreign. Sometimes drug com-

Table 4. Publication Aspects of Drug Handbooks

FULL NAME	SHORT NAME	AUTHOR(S) OR EDITOR(S)	PUBLISHER'S NAME AND ADDRESS	PRICE AS OF 1975
Accepted Dental Therapeutics	ADT	——	American Dental Association, 211 E. Chicago Ave., Chicago, Ill. 60611	$5.95
AMA Drug Evaluations	AMA-DE	——	Publishing Sciences Group, Inc., Acton, Mass. 01720	$22.00
American Drug Index	ADI	Charles O. Wilson and Tony E. Jones	J. B. Lippincott Co., E. Washington Sq., Philadelphia, Pa. 19105	$12.50
American Hospital Formulary Service	AHFS	Judith A. Kepler, Editor	American Society of Hospital Pharmacists, 4630 Montgomery Ave., Washington, D.C. 20014	$35.00 + $15.00/ year
American Druggist Blue Book	Blue Book	Stanley Siegelman, Editor	American Druggist, 224 W. 57th St., New York, N.Y. 10019	$7.00
Compendium of Pharmaceuticals and Specialties	Compendium or CPS	Gerald N. Rotenberg, Editor	The Canadian Pharmaceutical Association, 175 College St., Toronto, Ontario M5T 1P8, Canada	$15.00
Current Drug Handbook	Current Drug Handbook	Mary W. Falconer, H. Robert Patterson, and Edward A. Gustafson	W. B. Saunders Co., W. Washington Sq., Philadelphia, Pa.19105	$5.75
de Haen Nonproprietary Name Index	de Haen NNI	——	Paul de Haen, 11 W. 42nd St., New York, N.Y. 10036	$20.00
The United States Dispensatory	Dispensatory (U.S.)	Arthur Osol and Robertson Pratt	J. B. Lippincott Co., E. Washington Sq., Philadelphia, Pa. 19105	$30.00
Drugs of Choice	Drugs of Choice	Walter Modell, Editor	C. V. Mosby Co., 11830 Westline Dr. St. Louis, Mo. 63141	$23.75
Drugs in Current Use and New Drugs	Drugs in Current Use	Walter Modell, Editor	Springer Publishing Co., 200 Park Ave. S., New York, N.Y. 10003	$4.75
Extra Pharmacopoeia (Martindale) Incorporating Squire's Companion	EP or Martindale	Norman W. Blacow, Editor	Council of the Pharmaceutical Society of Great Britain, c/o Rittenhouse Book Distributors, 1706 Rittenhouse Sq., Philadelphia, Pa. 19103	$39.00

Table 4. Publication Aspects of Drug Handbooks (continued)

FULL NAME	SHORT NAME	AUTHOR(S) OR EDITOR(S)	PUBLISHER'S NAME AND ADDRESS	PRICE AS OF 1975
Facts and Comparisons	Facts and Comparisons	Erwin K. Kastrup, Editor	Facts and Comparisons, 1100 Oran Drive, St. Louis, Mo. 63137	$20.00 + $10.00/year
Handbook of Non-Prescription Drugs	HND	George B. Griffenhagen and Linda L. Hawkins, Co-editors	American Pharmaceutical Association, 2215 Constitution Ave., N.W., Washington, D.C. 20037	$7.50
Identification Guide for Tablets and Capsules	Identification Guide	R. C. Gupta and J. Kofoed	Canada Law Book Co. Ltd., 100 Richmond St. E., Toronto, Ontario, Canada	Out of print
Index Nominum	Index Nominum	H.-P. Jasperson	Centre Scientifique de la Société de Pharmacie, Zurich, c/o Drug Intelligence Publications, Dept. C-1, Hamilton Press, Hamilton, Ill. 62341	$65.75
International Nonproprietary Names for Pharmaceutical Substances: Cumulative List Number 3	INN	————	World Health Organization, c/o Q Corporation, 49 Sheridan Ave., Albany, N.Y. 12210	$10.80
Specifications for the Quality Control of Pharmaceutical Preparations; Second Edition of the International Pharmacopoeia	International Pharmacopoeia	————	World Health Organization, c/o Q Corporation, 49 Sheridan Ave., Albany, N.Y. 12210	$24.00 + $5.60/1971 Supplement
Isolation and Identification of Drugs in Pharmaceuticals, Body Fluids and Postmortem Material	Isolation and Identification of Drugs	E. G. C. Clarke	The Pharmaceutical Press, c/o Rittenhouse Book Distributors, 1706 Rittenhouse Sq., Philadelphia, Pa. 19103	Vol. 1, $39.00; Vol. 2, $32.40
Medical Letter on Drugs and Therapeutics	Medical Letter	————	The Medical Letter, 56 Harrison St., New Rochelle, N.Y. 10801	$19.50/year
Merck Index; an Encyclopedia of Chemicals and Drugs	Merck Index	Paul G. Stecher, Editor	Merck and Co., Inc., Rahway, N.J. 07065	$15.00
Modern Drug Encyclopedia and Therapeutic Index, and Modern Drugs, the Supplement to Modern Drug Encyclopedia	Modern Drug Encyclopedia	Arthur J. Lewis, Editor	The Yorke Medical Group, The Dun-Donnelley Publishing Corp., 666 Fifth Ave., New York, N.Y. 10019	$33.00

Table 4. Publication Aspects of Drug Handbooks (continued)

FULL NAME	SHORT NAME	AUTHOR(S) OR EDITOR(S)	PUBLISHER'S NAME AND ADDRESS	PRICE AS OF 1975
National Formulary	NF	———	Mack Publishing Co. 20th and Northampton St., Easton, Pa. 18042	$15.00
Organische-Chemische Arzneimittel und ihre Synonyma (eine internationale Übersicht)	*Negwer*	Martin Negwer	Akademie-Verlag, c/o Drug Intelligence Publications, Dept. C-1, Hamilton Press, Hamilton, Ill. 62341	$59.50
New Drugs, Evaluated by the A.M.A. Council on Drugs, 1967	*New Drugs*	———	American Medical Association, 535 N. Dearborn St., Chicago, Ill. 60610	Out of print
Pharmacological and Chemical Synonyms; a Collection of Names of Drugs and Other Compounds Drawn from the Medical Literature of the World	*Pharmacological and Chemical Synonyms*	E. E. J. Marler	International Publications Service, 114 E. 32nd St., New York, N.Y. 10016	$43.00
pharmIndex	*pharmIndex*	———	Skyline Publishers Inc., P.O. Box 1029, Portland, Oreg. 97207	$45.00 + $28.00/year
Physicians' Desk Reference and Supplements	PDR	Charles E. Baker, Jr., Publisher	Medical Economics, a subsidiary of Litton Publications, Oradell, N.J. 07649	$12.50 including Supplements
Drug Topics Red Book and Supplements	*Red Book*	Arthur Short	Topics Publishing Co., 550 Kinderkamack Road, Oradell, N.J. 07649	$15.00 including Supplements
USAN and the USP Dictionary of Drug Names and Supplements	USAN/USP-DDN	Mary C. Griffiths, Editor	United States Pharmacopeial Convention, Inc., 12601 Twinbrook Parkway, Rockville, Md. 20852	$18.50
The Pharmacopeia of the United States of America (The United States Pharmacopeia)	USP	———	Mack Publishing Co. 20th and Northampton St., Easton, Pa. 18042	$25.00

Table 4. Publication Aspects of Drug Handbooks (continued)

FULL NAME	SHORT NAME	AUTHOR(S) OR EDITOR(S)	PUBLISHER'S NAME AND ADDRESS	PRICE AS OF 1975
Unlisted Drugs and Unlisted Drugs Index-Guide 1971 and *Unlisted Drugs Index-Guide/III*	*UD* and *UD Index-Guide*	B. R. Anzlowar, Editor	Unlisted Drugs, Box 401, Chatham, N.J. 07928	$80.00/year; IG 1971, $125.00; IG/III, $290.00
Veterinarians' Blue Book and Therapeutic Index; a Scientifically Descriptive Listing of Veterinary Drugs, Biologicals and Foods, and Feed Additives of American Manufacturers	*Veterinarians' Blue Book*	Hadley C. Stephenson and Stanley G. Mittelstaedt	The Reuben H. Donnelley Corp., 466 Lexington Ave., New York, N.Y. 10017	Out of print

panies send out cards on their own drugs, and they are useful when kept in a card file. It isn't necessary to keep a single service filed by itself. All the information on one product can be kept in one place in the alphabet, whatever its source, as long as you have made the decision as to whether you are going to file by generic name or trade name. If you decide to use both, you must remember to look in more than one place or insert cross-reference cards from one name to the other. A well-maintained card file is the most current source of general information you can have, and it can be used quickly and easily while you are answering a question over the phone, but this convenience is paid for in the time it takes to file the cards when they come in. A misfiled card is information completely lost!

We have deliberately discussed cost in terms of your time in using the sources before we have called your attention to their prices, because books are the cheapest research tools you are likely to encounter. With handbooks, the cost in your time in using them, if they are inconvenient or too frequently fail to give you the information you need, will be far greater than the initial price of the handbook. When the choice is finally made, Table 4 should help you in ordering a book and paying for it.

CHAPTER 6

PART 2

PRIMARY SOURCES
INTRODUCTION

As the pharmacist's role changes, a multitude of original publications are increasing in importance to him and are challenging handbooks for their traditional central position. These publications are called "primary" to distinguish them from those which digest information from original sources and are called "secondary" or "tertiary," depending on the distance they are removed from the original report of a scientific experiment or clinical observation. Most of the questions posed about Farmlit in Chapter 2 can be answered in more detail by checking original papers, and some will not be answered adequately unless the primary publication is consulted.

The nature of his profession engenders problems for the pharmacist in the quality and quantity of the primary literature he uses. Since pharmacy stands at the borderline between the physical sciences, primarily chemistry, and the biological sciences, primarily medicine and preclinical sciences, the pharmacist is indeed in the maelstrom. On the one hand he is dealing with a healing art which is becoming more concerned with the whole person and the social responsibilities of the health professional, and on the other hand he is involved with a chemical entity which is becoming increasingly subjected to the control of the physical scientist's tools of measurement and analysis. Not only is the literature of interest to the pharmacist very extensive, but it is recorded and disseminated in different ways depending upon the particular discipline and function involved.

Table 5. Sources of More Extensive or More Specialized

AUTHOR(S)	TITLE	VIEWPOINT AND PURPOSE	GEOGRAPHIC SCOPE	DATE
Andrews, Theodora, and Marna Jo Young	The Literature of Pharmacognosy and Medicinal Chemistry	"A resource collection necessary for background information and on-going research in the study of medicinal compounds whether from naturally occurring materials or from laboratory syntheses." For libraries and reference	International	1972
Andrews, Theodora	Thesis Manual for Students in the Pharmaceutical Sciences	A description of abstracting and indexing sources for an extensive review on a thesis topic	American and foreign	1966
Andrews, Theodora, and J. Oslet	World List of Pharmacy Periodicals — revised and enlarged edition, 1975	A complete listing of all pharmacy periodicals known by the authors and drawn from many lists. For reference purposes	International	1975
Bloomfield, J. C.	Drug Information Sources. A bibliography — second edition	To "be used as a reference source by pharmacists engaged in general practice"	International. Arranged by country within each kind of source	1973
Brunn, Alice Lefler	How to Find Out in Pharmacy. A guide to sources of pharmaceutical information	An extensive selection for reference purposes. Bibliography and guide intended for students and practitioners	Primarily British and American	1969
de Haen, Paul, and Robert E. Pearson	Best Sources for Drug-Therapy Information	Primarily a description for physicians of quick sources of therapeutic information	U.S.	1973
Hellums, Betty Ann	A Manual to the Literature of Pharmacy	An extensive selection for reference purposes. Annotated bibliography	Primarily American	1968
Hirschman, Joseph L.	Building a Clinically-Oriented Drug Information Service	Contains a selected, classified list of Drug Information Service Reference Sources	Primarily U.S.	1972
Jackson, Elizabeth Christian	Books for Pharmacy Colleges 1962-1968. Part 1 and Part 2	Supplement to Zachert-Thomasson list, selected by editor and 9 consultants from faculties of colleges of pharmacy. Classified bibliography with index	Largely U.S.	1969

Bibliographies in Pharmacy and Allied Sciences

← GENERAL SCOPE, COVERAGE, AND LIMITATIONS	NAME AND ADDRESS OF SOURCE OR JOURNAL REFERENCE
Over 200 items listed as bibliographies, textbooks and monographs, dictionaries, etc., comprehensive works, reviews and annuals, abstracts and indexes, and periodicals	*American Journal of Pharmaceutical Education* 36:758-764, Dec. 1972
27 abstracting and indexing sources described in detail. Includes good sections on search method and bibliographic form and style	Librarian, Purdue University Pharmacy Library, Lafayette, Indiana 47907
1,940 titles, current and discontinued in "all aspects of pharmacy (formulation, retail, hospital, clinical, manufacturing, etc.) pharmacology, pharmacognosy, toxicology, and some related material in the soap, perfumery and cosmetics fields," drug abuse and alcoholism. Also provided are addresses of publishers, frequency and type of publication, sources in which indexed, and a geographic index	American Society of Hospital Pharmacists, 4630 Montgomery Ave., Washington, D.C. 20014. (Originally published in *American Journal of Hospital Pharmacy* 32:85-122, Jan. 1975)
A list of some 600 handbooks, dictionaries, and basic reference sources in pharmacy, pharmacology, and toxicology. No index. The first edition was an appendix to an excellent article, "Documentation in the pharmacy and its classification," *Pharmaceutical Journal* 206:20-22, Jan. 9, 1971, which covers British sources primarily	*Drug Intelligence and Clinical Pharmacy* 8:184-194, Apr. 1974. Originally published in *Pharmaceutische Zeitung* 118:1311-1322, Aug. 16, 1973
Contains some 400 references for general use as well as in pharmacy and related sciences. Lists pharmacy and medical libraries in the U.S. and Great Britain	Pergamon Press Inc., Maxwell House, Fairview Park, Elmsford, N.Y. 10523
Evaluates seven sources and lists 30 drug information centers	*Patient Care* 7:50-67, Feb. 1, 1973
Resource manual for pharmacy literature course covering some 300 general and pharmacy sources. Contains an introduction on library use	Department of Library Science, University of Mississippi, University, Mississippi 38677
79 selected, clinically oriented references, including a number of medical texts	In Francke, Donald E., and Harvey A. K. Whitney, Jr., editors *Perspectives in Clinical Pharmacy*. Hamilton Press, Inc., Hamilton, Ill. 62341. Pp. 150-177
1,163 texts and library materials for schools of pharmacy	American Association of Colleges of Pharmacy, 4630 Montgomery Ave., Washington, D.C. 20014. (Originally published in *American Journal of Pharmaceutical Education* 33:246-247, May 1969, and 411-458, Aug. 1969)

Table 5. Sources of More Extensive or More Specialized

AUTHOR(S)	TITLE	VIEWPOINT AND PURPOSE	GEOGRAPHIC SCOPE	DATE
King, Charles M., and Betty A. Hellums; Thudium, Vern F., and Robert E. Pearson	Drug Information Services: Two Operational Models	Contains lists of selected drug information sources for a drug information center, that at the University of Alabama (Model I). Model II (Michigan Regional Drug Information Network) is more fully described below	Primarily U.S.	1972
National Library of Medicine (Winifred Sewell)	Drug Literature. Report prepared for the study of "Interagency coordination in drug research and regulation" by the Subcommittee on Reorganization and International Organization of the Senate Committee on Government Operations	Subtitled "A factual survey on 'The nature and magnitude of the drug literature...'", it is addressed primarily to the Subcommittee. Discusses various kinds of literature in terms of those who produce and use it	Primarily U.S.	1963
Nemec, Dolores	The Pharmacist's Reference Shelf	Highly selective bibliography for pharmacist's personal collection or small community pharmacy. Annotated bibliography	U.S.	1972
Pasztor, Magda, and Jenny Hopkins	Bibliography of Pharmaceutical Reference Literature	An extensive selection for reference purposes. Annotated bibliography directed to teachers and librarians	Largely English language. United Kingdom viewpoint	1968
Pearson, Robert E., George L. Phillips, and Vern F. Thudium	Final Report, Project to Develop, Evaluate, and Demonstrate a Pilot Drug Information and Drug Therapy Analysis and Reporting System, University of Michigan Regional Drug Information Network	Contains lists of selected drug information sources for a drug information center and for satellites, as well as a bibliography of articles selected for a file in a drug information center	Primarily English language	1971

DRUG HANDBOOKS 49

Bibliographies in Pharmacy and Allied Sciences

GENERAL SCOPE, COVERAGE, AND LIMITATIONS	NAME AND ADDRESS OF SOURCE OR JOURNAL REFERENCE
250 sources listed in Appendix I, Basic Reference List (64) and Appendix K, Literature Information Services	Pharmacy-Related Program Branch, National Center for Health Services Research and Development, Health Services and Mental Health Administration, Public Health Service, Department of Health, Education, and Welfare, Rockville, Md. (For sale by Superintendent of Documents, DHEW Publication No. (HSM) 72-3030)
Lists of journals and drug information sources in appendices are largely supplanted now	Out of print. Text appeared in *American Journal of Hospital Pharmacy* 22:4-29, Jan. 1965
Basic reference sources in pharmacy plus other books to "be given priority in building a reference library." Includes publishers' addresses and costs. 52 items plus 12 on drug interactions	Librarian, F. B. Power Pharmaceutical Library, University of Wisconsin, Madison, Wis. 53706
Some 450 sources of general reference, general science, and pharmacy interest. Excellent annotations. Lists and describes many pertinent associations	Pharmaceutical Press, 17 Bloomsbury Square, London W.C. 1
23 sources for a satellite and approximately 250 for a drug information center. Over 1,000 references to journal articles arranged generally in order by the American Hospital Formulary Service classification scheme adapted	University of Michigan Hospital Pharmacy — University of Michigan College of Pharmacy, Ann Arbor, Michigan 48104

Table 5. Sources of More Extensive or More Specialized

AUTHOR(S)	TITLE	VIEWPOINT AND PURPOSE	GEOGRAPHIC SCOPE	DATE
Reilly, Mary Jo	Drug Information: Literature Review of Needs, Resources, and Services	A literature survey on drug information services, including special sections on resources for different audiences and appendices with publications lists	Primarily U.S.	1972
Sonnedecker, Glenn	The Pharmacist as a Book Collector	A guide to collecting especially in the history of pharmacy	International	1961
Special Libraries Association, Pharmaceutical Section, Science-Technology Division	Drug Information Sources: a World List	Annotated bibliography of handbooks containing information on drugs from throughout the world, primarily useful to libraries	International	1965
Walton, Charles A., Patricia Moynahan Mullins, and Ann B. Amerson	Drug Literature Utilization: Selection, Evaluation and Communication	Contains a select bibliography of reference works for a drug information service	Primarily U.S.	1972
Wilson, C. O.	Literature	Textual discussion of general sources, more for the organization than the individual	International	1970
Zachert, Martha Jane K., and C. Larry Thomasson	Bibliography of Books and Reference Works Relating to the Professional Courses in the Pharmaceutical Curriculum. Part 1 and Part 2	Recommendations of faculty of 43 colleges of pharmacy. Classified bibliography with index	Largely U.S.	1963

Bibliographies in Pharmacy and Allied Sciences

GENERAL SCOPE, COVERAGE, AND LIMITATIONS	NAME AND ADDRESS OF SOURCE OR JOURNAL REFERENCE
Separate lists and some discussion of types of sources and specific sources used by researchers, physicians, nurses and pharmacists. Appendix A lists names and addresses of researcher resources (46); Appendix B, Drug information sources (4); Appendix C, Drug information references commonly available in community and hospital pharmacies (18); Appendix D, Publications on drug interactions (6); Appendix E, Drug information reference sources (58)	Health Services and Mental Health Administration, Public Health Service, Department of Health, Education and Welfare, Rockville, Md. (For sale by Superintendent of Documents, DHEW Publication No. (HSM) 72-3013)
Incidentally lists a few prominent pharmacists, source books and collector's items	*American Journal of Hospital Pharmacy 18*:24-30, Jan. 1961
Over 150 separate handbooks from about 30 different countries, which "report for each drug its composition, variant names, actions, indications, dosage, manufacturer, supply and price."	Originally published in *American Journal of Pharmacy 129*:4-10, 59-64, 95-101, 128-134, 172-176, 211-216, 257-261, 303-306, and 372-377, 1957; and *ibid. 136*:52-70, 152-164, 257-267, 1964; *137*: 35-40, 69-81, 1965
32 reference works (handbooks and tests); 15 primary literature sources (periodicals); 12 secondary literature sources. Publishers' addresses appended. Bibliography of 113 references on drug information services and literature evaluation	In Blissitt, Charles W., O. Lynn Webb, and Walter F. Stanaszek, editors, *Clinical Pharmacy Practice*. Lea & Febiger, 600 S. Washington Square, Philadelphia, Pa. 19106. Pp. 347-406
Largely historical description of 150 sources such as pharmacopoeias and official compendia, handbooks and periodicals, with a selected list of books. Somewhat out of date	In Osol, A., editor, *Remington's Pharmaceutical Sciences*, 14th ed. Mack Publishing Co., Easton, Pa 18042. Pp.55-67
998 texts and library materials for schools of pharmacy	American Association of Colleges of Pharmacy, 4630 Montgomery Ave., Washington, D.C. 20014. (Originally published in *American Journal of Pharmaceutical Education 27*:266-290, Spring 1963, and 361-421, Summer 1963)

Table 5. Sources of More Extensive or More Specialized

MEDICINE

AUTHOR(S)	TITLE	VIEWPOINT AND PURPOSE	GEOGRAPHIC SCOPE	DATE
Brandon, Alfred N.	Selected List of Books and Journals for the Small Medical Library	Selection list for medical libraries. Classified bibliography	Primarily U.S.	1973
Inke, Gabor	A List of Most Frequently Recommended Medical Textbooks	Recommended listing based on responses to questionnaires to medical schools, containing lists of all current textbooks in 47 subjects representing disciplines in medical curriculum. Classified bibliography	U.S.	1971
Moll, Wilhelm	Basic Journal List for Small Hospital Libraries	A core periodical list for a very small hospital library based on a questionnaire to 23 physicians. Classified bibliography	U.S.	1969
Morton, Leslie T.	How to Use a Medical Library	A brief guide for medical practitioners, research workers, and medical librarianship trainees	British	1971
Stearns, Norman S., and Wendy W. Ratcliff	An Integrated Health-Science Core Library for Physicians, Nurses and Allied Health Practitioners in Community Hospitals	A list based on recommendations of 1,364 specialists, intended for a core collection library in a small hospital. Classified bibliography	U.S.	1970
Timour, John A.	Selected List of Journals for the Small Medical Library: a Comparative Analysis	An integration and comparison of periodical lists by Brandon, Stearns, and Moll, plus earlier ones. For a very small medical library. Classified bibliography	U.S.	1971

DRUG HANDBOOKS 53

Bibliographies in Pharmacy and Allied Sciences

← GENERAL SCOPE, COVERAGE, AND LIMITATIONS	NAME AND ADDRESS OF SOURCE OR JOURNAL REFERENCE
410 books and 136 periodicals in 50 subject fields. Contains an author index and an alphabetic list of journals. Contains a good bibliography of further sources and list of book dealers	*Bulletin of the Medical Library Association 61*: 179-200, Apr. 1973. Appears every two years in April
223 titles of which 94 are asterisked to indicate highest popularity	*Bulletin of the Medical Library Association 59*: 589-598, Oct. 1971
48 journals plus 22 supplementary ones	*Bulletin of the Medical Library Association 57*: 267-271, July 1969
Lists of principal indexes, book lists, bibliographies, catalogs, and abstracting services	William Heinemann Medical Books, 23 Bedford Square, London WC1B 3HT
A total of 104 books (including alternatives) and 74 periodicals, particularly useful for clinical pharmacy because of the list's clinical orientation. Also 19 items on a list of "Suggested reference materials for an integrated health-science core library"	*New England Journal of Medicine 283*: 1489-1498, Dec. 31, 1970
A total of 91 titles listed as highest rated (45) and next highest rated (46) in terms of inclusion and ranking on the various other lists. Within the two groups, there is a subject breakdown	*Bulletin of the Medical Library Association 59*: 87-93, Jan. 1971

Table 5. Sources of More Extensive or More Specialized

AUTHOR(S)	TITLE	VIEWPOINT AND PURPOSE	GEOGRAPHIC SCOPE	DATE
BIOLOGY				
Bottle, R. T., and H. V. Wyatt, editors	The Use of Biological Literature. 2nd ed.	A textbook with bibliographies. Intended for use by librarians and scientists and in particular "to plan courses for undergraduate and postgraduate students..."	Primarily British and U.S.	1971
Council of Biology Editors. Committee on Form and Style	CBE Style Manual. 3rd ed.	A style manual with excellent bibliographies	U.S. and international	1972
Kerker, Ann E., and Henry T. Murphy	Biological and Biomedical Resource Literature	A selected list of literature resources directed to research investigators, students, and librarians	Primarily U.S.	1968
Smith, Roger C., and W. Malcolm Reid	Guide to the Literature of the Life Sciences. 8th ed.	Textbook with bibliographies. Intended for use by students, teachers, and specialists	U.S. viewpoint; many European sources	1972
CHEMISTRY				
American Chemical Society	Literature of Chemical Technology (Advances in Chemistry Series 78)	Results of a symposium surveying a wide variety of chemical industries	U.S. and European	1968
Bottle, R. T.	The Use of the Chemical Literature. 2nd ed.	Textbook with bibliographic and reference material for introducing the chemistry student to the literature	European and U.S.	1969
Burman, C. R.	How to Find Out in Chemistry	Textbook and career guide	European and U.S.	1965
Mellon, M. G.	Chemical Publications. Their Nature and Use. 4th ed.	Textbook with bibliographies, for introducing the student to the literature	U.S. and European	1965

Bibliographies in Pharmacy and Allied Sciences

GENERAL SCOPE, COVERAGE, AND LIMITATIONS	NAME AND ADDRESS OF SOURCE OR JOURNAL REFERENCE
Covers all of biology including botany, zoology, ecology, genetics, biochemistry, and biophysics and some biomedical aspects. Includes such special kinds of publication as theses, patents, and instruments and equipment catalogs	Archon Books, The Shoe String Press, 995 Sherman Ave., Hamden, Conn. 06514
Section on Style in Special Fields contains bibliographies related to standard terminology, classification, etc. Annotated bibliography at end lists other style manuals, etc., dictionaries and source books, indexes and periodical lists, standards and codes, handbooks, zoological nomenclature, and botanical and microbiological nomenclature	American Institute of Biological Sciences, 3900 Wisconsin Ave., N.W., Washington, D.C. 20016
Annotated lists of various kinds of reference material plus bibliography only for fifteen different broad subjects. An extensive selection	Purdue Research Foundation, Lafayette, Ind.
Originally for zoological sciences. Particularly good for taxonomic sources. Also has section on library. Around 1500 references	Burgess Publishing Co., 426 S. Sixth St., Minneapolis, Minn. 55415

Most pertinent chapter is by Howard T. Bonnett, "The literature of pharmaceutical and medicinal chemistry," pp. 152-190. A brief introduction is followed by over 1,000 references	American Chemical Society, 1155 Sixteenth St., N.W., Washington, D.C. 20036
Discussion of sources by type and subject with chapters on standard tables of physical data, patents, and government and trade publications	Archon Books, The Shoe String Press, 995 Sherman Ave., Hamden, Conn. 06514
Similar to text by Bottle, above, but older	Pergamon Press Inc., Maxwell House, Fairview Park, Elmsford, N.Y. 10523
Discussion of sources by type, with extensive discussions of patents and documents as well as the more usual primary, secondary, and tertiary publications	McGraw-Hill Book Co., 1221 Ave. of the Americas, New York, N.Y. 10020

In fact, if a pharmacist is to be thorough, he would do well to seek out not one but three guides to the literature: one for medicine, one for chemistry, and one for pharmacy. He also has need for the literature of sociology and economics and biology in general, particularly since pharmacognosy is still closely related to botany. With the changing concepts of pharmacy, the literature in the other fields assumes at least equal importance with that in the core of pharmacy. For this reason, we have chosen to cover all areas superficially, rather than to concentrate on a strict, traditional definition of pharmacy. The lists of further sources included in Table 5 will allow you to get additional detail in specific disciplines.

Our broad coverage requires that we be highly selective in the sources mentioned and described. Instead of presenting many titles, we shall enumerate characteristics of various kinds of publication and provide a few examples to show the influence of individual disciplines on similarities and differences between specific publications. Then we shall try to help you in your selection of materials for a personal collection or for use in response to a specific need.

Insofar as we evaluate individual items — either implicitly by selecting them for mention or explicitly by describing their advantages and disadvantages — we shall be following the general principles set forth in the section on handbooks, looking at their authority, purpose, scope and coverage, and special features which make them more useful than others. Other principles for evaluation of materials are touched on in Chapter 20.

CHAPTER 7

PERIODICALS

The first periodical reported individual research. Henry Oldenberg, of Bremen and London, recognized the need to record scientific progress when he persuaded his friends to send him letters reporting their observations. The resulting *Philosophical Transactions of the Royal Society*, which represented the beginning of journal publication in 1664, also began a memory for modern science. Books had, of course, been published earlier but, by definition, the periodical appears on a continuing basis, assuring the ongoing dissemination of new observations. If one gives a paper at a meeting today, it will have an effect on the audience, and may be reflected indirectly in later work by those who heard it, but the impact will not be nearly so great as if it is also published in a journal and becomes a part of the cumulative record.

Journals on physical science — such as the *Journal of Organic Chemistry* or the *Journal of the American Chemical Society* — have continued the tradition of reporting observations almost exclusively. Separate publications — for example, *Chemical and Engineering News, Chemical Week*, or *Chemistry and Industry* — report the "news" of the physical sciences; and yet others — for instance *Fortschritte der Medizinische Chemie* and *Chemical Reviews* — review the state of current progress in a given subject. Finally, there may be separate periodicals which publish brief communications or letters, such as *Tetrahedron Letters* and *Bio-*

chemical and Biophysical Research Communications. Such letters are also sometimes found in regular scientific journals.

In the field of medicine, on the other hand, one journal is apt to perform all of the aforementioned functions. The *Journal of the American Medical Association (JAMA)* and the *New England Journal of Medicine* supplement original articles with editorials which comment on and evaluate them. There are also special articles which may be reviews or may report experience rather than scientific observations. In these and other general medical journals, there are also "Letters to the Editor," news, book reviews, and a form particularly indigenous to medicine, the "rounds" type of presentation, which is a sort of esoteric puzzle page. The physician reader is invited to read a record of observations and laboratory findings for a particular patient and to diagnose the illness himself before reading on to find the final diagnosis, often determined after a pathological study postmortem. Some journals contain pictorial information, such as "Electrocardiograms of the Month" *(New York State Journal of Medicine)* for the physician to interpret.

In the various medical specialties, there are many journals that contain information on drugs. Particularly important is the *Annals of Internal Medicine.* There are also *Archives of Internal Medicine, American Journal of Medicine, American Journal of Obstetrics and Gynecology, American Journal of Diseases of Children, Pediatrics, Journal of Pediatrics, Journal of Urology, Anesthesia and Analgesia: Current Researches, Anesthesiology, British Journal of Anaesthesia, American Journal of Clinical Pathology, Journal of Clinical Pathology, Cancer Research, Cancer Chemotherapy Reports, Journal of the National Cancer Institute, Journal of Experimental Medicine, Proceedings of the Society of Experimental Biology and Medicine,* and *Proceedings of the Royal Society of Medicine,* to name but a few that are known to have many articles on drugs and their applications.

Between the chemical field and the medical field, there are the "preclinical sciences," ranging from biochemistry and biophysics to microbiology. Examples of journals of particular interest to pharmacists are: *Endocrinology, Virology, Journal of Bacteriology, Applied Microbiology, American Journal of Physiology,* and *Journal of Medicinal Chemistry.*

At the other end of the spectrum, there are the social sciences, which have a still different form of literature, because of the need to create a science from "soft data." Some journals in this area which the pharmacist may sometimes find useful include: *Medical Care Reviews, Journal of Health and Social Behavior, Medical Care, Inquiry, Milbank Memorial Fund Quarterly,* and *Social Work.*

In both the biological and the social sciences, one will find different types of journal depending on whether the information is addressed to research scientists or to practitioners. For the former, the pure science journal format of chemistry is apt to prevail, whereas for the latter, the applied science type, as exemplified by general medical periodicals, will be found. If you recognize the difference, you may save time in selecting those of interest.

Similarly, journals in the field of pharmacy vary from strictly original article research publications — such as *Journal of Pharmaceutical Sciences* and *Journal of Pharmacy and Pharmacology* — to *Drug Intelligence and Clinical Pharmacy* and *American Journal of Hospital Pharmacy,* whose coverage is more general because they are directed to the pharmacy practitioner.

The student soon learns which are the better periodicals as he learns to separate the wheat from the chaff in his scientific reading. He may not realize that one reason for some of the differences in quality is the "review process" or "peer review." When you submit a paper to an American scientific journal, in most cases it will be sent to one or more authorities on the subject of the paper, who will evaluate it for the editor. It may be returned to you for modification to conform with reviewers' suggestions. This process assures that the final publication will be of the quality set by the editorial board of the periodical and recognized by its readers.

One reason for the existence of such magazines as *Tetrahedron Letters* or *Biochemical and Biophysical Research Communications* is the occasional need of scientists to have their experiments reported quickly. These publications reprint typewritten material and truncate the review process so that primary responsibility for the quality and originality of the article rests with the author. In using papers from such sources, you should keep this limitation in mind.

Beware of journals which announce that they are designed for prompt publication since such statements can mean that the review process is minimal or nonexistent. Two such journals of pharmaceutical interest — *Current Therapeutic Research* and *Journal of Clinical Pharmacology* (formerly *Journal of New Drugs*) — publish many papers supported directly or indirectly by the pharmaceutical industry. They are a source of prompt information on new drugs, but some objectivity may be sacrificed to gain an article's timeliness.

The pharmacist is concerned about the quantity and accuracy of advertising in the serials he reads, but he may not have thought about the effect of the advertising revenue on the existence of the publication. In an editorial, Provost[1] says there are at least sixty-eight regional, state and local pharmaceutical publications in the United States. The majority "are state journals published under the auspices of state pharmaceutical associations." With the exception of "a few such journals, emanating from populous states with progressive state associations," these journals often reprint articles that have been published in national periodicals. Or they may "rarely or never publish any authored articles, neither original nor reprinted. A typical issue will contain (in addition to advertising, of course) a few news items based on news releases issued by pharmaceutical associations and governmental agencies, notices of transfer of ownership of community pharmacies, names of pharmacists who have been licensed in the state by reciprocity, and a few classified ads and obituaries — in short, nothing that could not be communicated more quickly, easily and economically via a newsletter."[1] Provost points out that, "in view of the decline in advertising being experienced by many journals in pharmacy" it is possible that "some state journals are being subsidized by association membership dues which might be better spent on other activities."[1]

Many state medical journals have also been perpetuated through advertising support. There are some, however, in which important original papers appear. *New York State Journal of Medicine,* and the regional journals, *New England Journal of Medicine, Southern Medical Journal,* and *Western Journal of Medicine,* formerly *California Medicine,* are all useful sources.

There is a continuing argument as to whether a periodical can maintain an editorial policy completely independent of influence from its advertisers. In my observation, the danger of sustaining bad publications by advertisers has been greater than that of subverting good ones.

To guide the pharmacist to some of the serials he will wish

to see regularly, a few key journals are arranged according to various kinds of pharmacy practice in the following lists. Official journals of professional societies will be received as a benefit of society membership.

General

Canadian Pharmaceutical Journal (Canadian Pharmaceutical Association)
FDA Drug Bulletin
FDA Papers
Journal of the American Pharmaceutical Association (The news and general interest publication of the Association)
Journal Mondial de Pharmacie (The official publication of the International Federation of Pharmacy, mostly in English)
Medical Letter on Drugs and Therapeutics (See Tables 1-4)
A general science magazine such as: *Science, Nature, BioScience, American Scientist, Scientific American*

Community Pharmacy

American Druggist
Chain Store Age, Drug Executives Edition and/or Drug Managers Edition
Drug Topics
NARD Journal (National Association of Retail Druggists)
Pharmacy Times
Voice of the Pharmacist (American College of Apothecaries)
Weekly Pharmacy Reports (The "Green Sheet")

Institutional Pharmacy

American Journal of Hospital Pharmacy (American Society of Hospital Pharmacists)
Canadian Journal of Hospital Pharmacy (Canadian Society of Hospital Pharmacists)
Hospital Pharmacy (Lippincott's) (See also *Hospital Pharmacy*, The "White Sheet," discussed in Chapter 9)

Hospital Progress (Catholic Hospital Association)
Hospitals (American Hospital Association)
Modern Hospital

Clinical Pharmacy

Annals of Internal Medicine (American College of Physicians)
British Medical Journal (British Medical Association)
Clinical Pediatrics
Clinical Pharmacology and Therapeutics (American Society for Pharmacology and Experimental Therapeutics)
Clinical Toxicology (American Academy of Clinical Toxicology)
DM: Disease-A-Month
Drug Intelligence and Clinical Pharmacy
Journal of the American Medical Association (JAMA)
Lancet
Medical Clinics of North America
New England Journal of Medicine (Massachusetts Medical Society)
Rational Drug Therapy, formerly *Pharmacology for the Physician* (American Society for Pharmacology and Experimental Therapeutics)

Industrial Pharmacy

American Perfumer and Cosmetics
Drug and Cosmetic Industry
F-D-C Reports (The "Pink Sheet")
Oil, Paint and Drug Reporter
Product Management, for the Drug, Cosmetic and Allied Industries, formerly *Drug Trade News*

Research Pharmacy

(Physical Pharmacy, Pharmaceutical Chemistry, Pharmacology, etc.)
Biochemical Pharmacology
British Journal of Pharmacology (British Pharmacological Society)
Drug Research Reports (The "Blue Sheet")
Drugs
Japanese Journal of Pharmacology (in English; Japanese Pharmacological Society)

Journal of Medicinal Chemistry (American Chemical Society)
Journal of Natural Products, formerly *Lloydia* (American Society of Pharmacognosy)
Journal of Pharmaceutical Sciences (American Pharmaceutical Association)
Journal of Pharmacology and Experimental Therapeutics (American Society for Pharmacology and Experimental Therapeutics)
Journal of Pharmacy and Pharmacology (Pharmaceutical Society of Great Britain)
Molecular Pharmacology (American Society for Pharmacology and Experimental Therapeutics)
Neuropharmacology
Pharmacological Reviews (American Society for Pharmacology and Experimental Therapeutics)
Toxicology and Applied Pharmacology (Society of Toxicology)

Analytical Pharmacy and Clinical Chemistry

Clinical Chemistry (American Association of Clinical Chemists)
Journal of Laboratory and Clinical Medicine (Central Society for Clinical Research)
Scandinavian Journal of Clinical and Laboratory Investigation (Scandinavian Society for Clinical Chemistry and Clinical Physiology)

Miscellaneous

American Journal of Pharmaceutical Education (American Association of Colleges of Pharmacy)
Drug Information Journal, formerly *Drug Information Bulletin* (Drug Information Association)
Food, Drug, Cosmetic Law Reporter (Commerce Clearinghouse)
Pharmacy in History (American Institute of the History of Pharmacy)

Within the realm of pharmacy there are two special kinds of periodical that the pharmacist should not forget. The house organ, issued by manufacturers for physicians, pharmacists or other health professionals is mentioned in Chapter 9. The other special variety of publication is one that the pharmacist himself may issue. It is the newsletter distributed by a hospital or clinical pharmacist to keep associated health professionals informed of new developments in medication practices locally and new information on drugs in general. Though newsletters differ considerably among hospitals, many practicing hospital pharmacists find them useful communication mechanisms. A community pharmacist of my acquaintance provides a newsletter for his customers to inform them of good health practices.

How to Find Periodical Titles of Interest

Because of the broad scope of pharmacy, the number of pertinent scientific articles published annually can be estimated as between 150,000 and 200,000.[2] Whether or not this number is correct, even one percent of the total is probably more than a single individual can read. Yet if he is to remain abreast of his profession, he must have some kind of continual access to everything that is pertinent to the work he is doing. The answer is for him to read a few key journals regularly, and to find pertinent current titles from other sources with the assistance of abstracts, reviews, journal contents lists, or an alerting service.

For reading intensively, you will wish to subscribe to a few of the journals just listed and possibly some in special subject areas which can be located through the guides listed in Table 5. There are also library studies, which show the journals most popular at various institutions,[3] and citation studies, which enumerate journals most frequently cited by scientific authors.[4]

Such guides are usually not needed, however. It is a simple matter to determine which journals occur most frequently in bibliographies or footnotes of papers you are reading or in lists of articles in your field of interest. Examples of such lists are bibliographies from a search of MEDLINE (see Chapters 13 and 16) or the selected bibliographies which appear in journals like *American Journal of Hospital Pharmacy* and *Drug Intelligence & Clinical Pharmacy.*

Methods of keeping abreast of your current interests in journals you don't see regularly as well as becoming aware of periodicals to which you may wish to subscribe are: (1) reading abstracting publications such as *Medical Letter* or *ClinAlert* or sections of *International Pharmaceutical Abstracts* (e.g., "Drug Analysis," "Pharmacy Practice," "Investigational Drugs," or "Sociology, Economics and Ethics." (See Chapter 13); (2) scanning reviews (See Chapter 15); or (3) regular examination of the contents pages of hundreds of journals which are found in *Current Contents/Life Sciences* or *Current Contents/Clinical Practice*.

There are also series of *Current Contents* in Physical and Chemical Sciences and Social and Behavioral Sciences. *Current Contents* is simply a compilation of reproductions of the contents pages of journals. If you wish to read an article, you will have to find it elsewhere. *Current Contents* does give you the address of authors so that you may write for a reprint. Some sections, including those on Clinical Practice and Life Sciences, have keyword indexes which enable you to check each week for certain topics.

If one works for an organization that will invest in computerized or manual SDI services, or has regular access to a computer data base such as that in MEDLINE, he can get regularly updated listings covering his interests. "SDI" is an acronym for "selective dissemination of information" and describes the method by which the computer regularly selects from a broader data base only those references which fit a previously defined interest profile for a given individual. In this manner, one can obtain the relatively few references of greatest importance to a specific interest taken from several hundred or even several thousand journals each month.

References

1. Provost, George P. "State Pharmaceutical Journals: Legitimate Need or Ego Fulfillment." *American Journal of Hospital Pharmacy* 28:153, March 1971.

2. See pages 14 and 15 and Appendix A — Item 1 of National Library of Medicine, *Drug Literature* (cited in Table 5). Subsequently the author worked with a computer search of a month's file to find how many articles were indexed with at least one term for a drug or a chemical. We also did a sampling check of a few hundred journal issues. In each case, we found that about one-third of the articles contained information on drugs, although these articles appeared in roughly two-thirds of the journals. This meant that approximately 60,000-70,000 original articles on drugs were drawn each year from the 2,300 medical journals indexed at the National Library of Medicine.

3. See, for example, Wood, D. N. and Bower, C. A. "The Use of Biomedical Periodical Literature at the National Lending Library for Science and Technology." *Methods of Information in Medicine* 9:46-53, Jan. 1970; or Lasslo, Andrew. "An Estimate of Comparative Serial Literature Resources Supporting Research in Medicinal and Pharmaceutical

Chemistry in Major Libraries of the United States." *Bulletin of the Medical Library Association* 50:70-88, Jan. 1962.

    4. Garfield, Eugene. "Citation Analysis as a Tool in Journal Evaluation." *Science* 178:471-479, Nov. 3, 1972.

CHAPTER 8

BOOKS

Books are here defined as textbooks, specialized monographs or symposia on a special subject, or any publication of substantial size available generally from a commercial publisher. They differ from a periodical in that they are published just once. If they are popular, a new edition may be brought out, containing new material, but it will generally repeat most of the information that was in the former edition.

In contrast with periodicals — where characteristics of a research science journal differ from those of one in applied science in predictable ways — books can vary widely within any given subject and for whatever audience they are intended. Most reliable books have good indexes and are comprehensive, accurate, and up-to-date in the subject they cover. But the manners of presentation and organization are individual, and there may be a single author, several authors for the whole text, or different authors for each chapter.

The following discussion of interesting books in specific areas is, at best, a sampling and can give you only a flavor of what is available. To use a familiar analogy, it represents the tip of an iceberg. To gain a better idea of just how large the iceberg is, you may wish to look at Table 5 and some of the booklists cited therein. Table 5 itself does not list nearly every source guide available. Many of the bibliographies contained are updated frequently, so that you can use later editions to keep up to date.

In addition, current professional journals, such as *American Journal of Hospital Pharmacy, Drug Intelligence & Clinical Pharmacy, Journal of the American Pharmaceutical Association,* and *American Journal of Pharmaceutical Education,* list or review the most important new books in pharmacy and related fields as well as other materials, such as pamphlets and government publications.

In checking booklists, the pharmacist should be alert to titles which may mislead him to expect a coordinated text, when in fact the publication reports an original symposium or proceedings of a meeting in which there is little integration among the papers. The original papers may be excellent and well worth reading, as one would read a journal article, but they will not serve as basic texts except for very advanced study. One example of such publications is: Tedeschi, D. H. and Tedeschi, R. E., *Importance of Fundamental Principles in Drug Evaluation* (Raven Press, New York, 1968), the proceedings of a symposium held by the Section on Pharmacology and Biochemistry, Academy of Pharmaceutical Sciences, American Pharmaceutical Association, in May 1968. Another example is: *The Problems of Species Difference and Statistics in Toxicology,* edited by S. B. de C. Baker et al. (Excerpta Medica Foundation, Amsterdam, 1970), the proceedings of the European Society for the Study of Drug Toxicity meeting held March-April 1969 in Venice.

Books on Pharmacy

You will want to keep certain useful undergraduate texts in your collection. Books you will purchase will depend somewhat on the particular specialty you pursue. *The Pharmacist's Reference Shelf,* by Dolores Nemec (see Table 5), is a generally helpful guide to books you may wish to own. In addition to listing drug handbooks such as the ones described in Tables 1-4, she includes the following more general books in pharmacy:

Remington's Pharmaceutical Sciences. 15th ed. Mack Publishing Co., 20th and Northampton St., Easton, Pa. 18042, 1975. $35.00.

Coleman, Thomas E.
Profitable Drugstore Management. Prentice-Hall, Englewood Cliffs, N.J. 07632, 1970. $19.95.

How to Promote Your Retail Pharmacy; A Guide to Publicity, Advertising, Promotion. National Association of Retail Druggists, One E. Wacker Dr., Chicago, Ill. 60601, 1969. $5.00 (members, $4.00).

Keller, Bernard G., Jr. and Mickey C. Smith. *Pharmaceutical Marketing; An Anthology and Bibliography.* Williams & Wilkins Co., 428 E. Preston St., Baltimore, Md. 21202, 1969. $13.50.

Martin, Eric W., editor
Husa's Dispensing of Medication. 7th ed. Mack Publishing Co., 20th and Northampton St., Easton, Pa. 18042, 1971. $19.00. (Formerly *Husa's Pharmaceutical Dispensing.*)

or

Sprowls, Joseph B., editor
Prescription Pharmacy. 2nd ed. J. B. Lippincott Co., E. Washington Sq., Philadelphia, Pa. 19105, 1970. $18.00.

Bradley, Willis T., Carroll B. Gustafson and
Stoklosa J. Mitchell
Pharmaceutical Calculations. 5th ed. Lea and Febiger, Washington Sq., Philadelphia, Pa. 19106, 1968. $7.50

Claus, Edward P., Varro E. Tyler, Jr. and Lynn R. Brady
Pharmacognosy. 6th ed. Lea and Febiger, Washington Sq., Philadelphia, Pa. 19106, 1970. $17.50.

Lawrence, Carl A. and Seymour S. Block, editors
Disinfection, Sterilization and Preservation. Lea and Febiger, Washington Sq., Philadelphia, Pa. 19106, 1968. $30.00.

Sonnedecker, Glenn, reviser
Kremers and Urdang's History of Pharmacy. 3rd ed. J. B. Lippincott Co., E. Washington Sq., Philadelphia, Pa. 19105, 1963. $10.50.

Hassan, William E., Jr.
Law for the Pharmacy Student. Lea and Febiger, Washington Sq., Philadelphia, Pa. 19106, 1971. $11.50.

To supplement this basic law text, the pharmacist will also want the state laws affecting pharmacy for those states in which he is registered to practice and the "Federal Food, Drug and

Cosmetic Act and General Regulations for its Enforcement," and "Drug Abuse Control Amendments."

To add to this minimum collection in pharmacy, one can turn to "Bibliography of Books and Reference Works relating to the Professional Courses in the Pharmaceutical Curriculum," by Martha Jane K. Zachert and C. Larry Thomasson and to its supplement, "Books for Pharmacy Colleges, 1962-1968," by Elizabeth Christian Jackson (See Table 5). These bibliographies list hundreds of books which should be in the pharmacy college library, but which one would not wish to include in a private collection. They do provide an excellent starting point for selecting materials in an area of special interest.

If the pharmacist is to communicate effectively with his clientele, he should be aware of books about drugs for the layman. The American Pharmaceutical Association has prepared a four-page mimeographed "Popular and Semi-Popular Reading List on Drugs."

Books on Pharmacology and Related Subjects

Sometimes a question of the type asked in Chapter 3 — for instance, concerning the use of Farmlit when a patient is receiving insulin or the rapidity of its metabolism — will be better answered by a textbook or journal article than by a handbook. Textbooks in pharmacology and toxicology will usually be the first place to turn.

We have separated pharmacology and toxicology books from the pharmacy texts because it is in this area that the pharmacist's interest and information is expanding and changing at such a rate that it is as difficult to pin down a selection of books as it is to isolate a point in time when one can sum up man's knowledge on the mode of action of his medications and say, "This is it!" Such terms as "clinical pharmacy" and "clinical pharmacology," "biopharmaceutics" and "pharmacokinetics," all relate to a changing depth of knowledge and concern with what actually happens in the individual when the drug and the human organism interact. Similarly, the mounting concern with adverse reactions, poisonings, drug interactions, and the physiologic aspects of drug abuse lead to new varieties of publication in the broad area of toxicology.

L. S. Goodman and A. Gilman's *The Pharmacological Basis*

of Therapeutics (5th ed., Macmillan Publishing Co., 866 Third Ave., New York, N.Y. 10022, 1975, $30.00) is still the best reference source in pharmacology. Nemec also lists the very useful:

Aviado, Domingo M.
Krantz and Carr's Pharmacologic Principles of Medical Practice. 8th ed. Williams & Wilkins Co., 428 E. Preston St., Baltimore, Md. 21202, 1972. $24.50.

Cutting, Windsor C.
Handbook of Pharmacology. 5th ed. Appleton-Century-Crofts, 440 Park Ave. S., New York, N.Y. 10016, 1972. $11.50.

Other recent sources of interest are:

Goldstein, Avram, Lewis Aronow and Sumner M. Kalman
Principles of Drug Action: The Basis of Pharmacology. 2nd ed. Harper & Row, Scranton, Pa. 18512, 1974. $21.50.

La Du, Bert N., H. George Mandel and
E. Leong Way, editors
Fundamentals of Drug Metabolism and Disposition. Williams & Wilkins Co., 428 E. Preston St., Baltimore, Md. 21202, 1971. $21.75.

There is also an excellent French language review on metabolism of individual drugs which has pertinence in our thinking about various areas of pharmacology. The second volume of a projected five volume series is scheduled for release in 1975.

Hirtz, J.
The Fate of Drugs in the Organism. Bibliography and analytical tables prepared by a working group of the Société de Technique Pharmaceutique under the chairmanship of J. Hirtz. Volume 1, Bibliography and Tables. Marcel Dekker, New York and Drug Intelligence Publications, Dept. C-1, Hamilton, Ill. 62341, 1970. $65.25. Volume II 1975. $59.50.

Some interesting and useful sources covering the newer concepts in pharmacology include the following:

BIOPHARMACEUTICS AND PHARMACOKINETICS

Wagner, John G.
Fundamentals of Clinical Pharmacokinetics. Drug Intelli-

gence Publications, Dept. C-1, Hamilton, Ill. 62341, 1975. $37.50.

Gibaldi, Milo and Donald Perrier
Pharmacokinetics. Marcel Dekker, 270 Madison Ave., New York, N. Y. 10016, 1975. $19.50

Notari, Robert E.
Biopharmaceutics and Pharmacokinetics; An Introduction. 2nd ed. Marcel Dekker, 270 Madison Ave., New York, N. Y. 10016, 1975. $13.75.

Ritschel, W. A.
Handbook of Basic Pharmacokinetics. Drug Intelligence Publications, Dept. C-1, Hamilton, Ill. 62341, 1976. $16.00.

Curry, Stephen H.
Drug Disposition and Pharmacokinetics — with a Consideration of Pharmacological and Clinical Relationships. Blackwell Scientific Publications, c/o J. B. Lippincott, E. Washington Sq., Philadelphia, Pa. 19105, 1974. $17.50.

Swarbrick, James, editor
Current Concepts in the Pharmaceutical Sciences: Dosage Form Design and Bioavailability. Lea & Febiger, Washington Sq., Philadelphia, Pa. 19106, 1973. $19.50.

Wagner, John G.
Biopharmaceutics and Relevant Pharmacokinetics, with a Special Chapter on "Quality Control" by M. Pernarowski. Drug Intelligence Publications, Dept. C-1, Hamilton, Ill., 62341, 1971. $15.00.

One should also check the July issue of the *Journal of Pharmaceutical Sciences* which includes a section entitled "Biopharmaceutics" in its annual review of publications in "Pharmaceutical Sciences: Literature Review of Pharmaceutics."

CLINICAL PHARMACY AND CLINICAL PHARMACOLOGY

Melmon, Kenneth L. and Howard F. Morrelli, editors
Clinical Pharmacology; Basic Principles in Therapeutics.

Macmillan Publishing Co., 866 Third Ave., New York, N.Y. 10022, 1972. $16.00; paper, $11.95.

Francke, Donald E. and Whitney, Harvey A. K., Jr., editors
Perspectives in Clinical Pharmacy. Drug Intelligence Publications, Dept. C-1, Hamilton Press, Hamilton, Ill. 62341, 1972. $15.00.

Blissitt, Charles W., O. Lynn Webb and Walter F. Stanaszek, editors
Clinical Pharmacy Practice. Lea and Febiger, Washington Sq., Philadelphia, Pa. 19106, 1972. $19.50.

Smith, William E.
Clinical Pharmacy Services in a Community Hospital. DHEW Pub. No. HSM 72-3019. Prepared for: Drug Related Studies, National Center for Health Services Research and Development, HSMHA, Department of Health, Education, and Welfare. Government Printing Office, Washington, D.C., January 1972.

Knoben, James E., Philip O. Anderson and
Arthur S. Watanabe, editors
Handbook of Clinical Drug Data. 3rd ed. Drug Intelligence Publications, Dept. C-1, Hamilton Press, Hamilton, Ill. 62341, 1973. $4.75.

For two special areas of particular interest in clinical pharmacy, the following publications are of importance:

Shirkey, Harry C.
Pediatric Dosage Handbook, 1973. American Pharmaceutical Association, 2215 Constitution Ave., N.W., Washington, D.C. 20037, 1973. $2.00.

Francke, Donald E.
Handbook of I.V. Additive Reviews, 1971. Drug Intelligence Publications, Dept. C-1, Hamilton Press, Hamilton, Ill. 62341, 1971. $3.75. (1970, 1972 and 1973 *Handbooks.* $3.75.)

Books on Toxicology and Associated Disciplines

The books at the core of toxicology fall into three overlapping areas: identification of what is in compounds such as household chemicals; identification of the toxicant in the body; and discussions of toxic levels, antidotes, and therapy.

For identification of what is in the compound, two sources are generally recognized:

Gleason, Marion N., Robert E. Gosselin, Harold C. Hodge and Roger P. Smith
Clinical Toxicology of Commercial Products. 3rd ed. Williams & Wilkins Co., 428 E. Preston St., Baltimore, Md. 21202, 1969. $27.00.

Poison Cards. National Clearinghouse for Poison Control Centers, 5401 Westbard Ave., Bethesda, Md. 20014.

A very new service which appears to be extremely useful has been introduced by Poisindex, Inc. (National Center for Poison Information, Rocky Mountain Poison Center, 8th and Cherokee, Denver, Colo. 80204). It is a microfiche listing of the ingredients of many thousands of commercial products, complemented by a separate index of 200 different managements. Quarterly updating is scheduled. The annual subscription of around $1,000 may make it available only through poison information centers.

For the industrial toxicologist, there are a number of other identification references which may also be useful in a Poison Information Center:

Manufacturing Chemist's Association
Data Sheets (on chemicals ranging from acetaldehyde to zirconium, available at 50 cents each) and *Safety Guides* (on such topics as "Disposal of Hazardous Waste" (SG-9), available for 25 cents each). Manufacturing Chemist's Association, 1825 Connecticut Ave., N.W., Washington, D.C. 20009.

Sax, N. Irving
Dangerous Properties of Industrial Materials. 4th ed. Van Nostrand Reinhold, 450 W. 33rd St., New York, N.Y. 10001, 1975. $42.50.

Elkins, H. B.
Chemistry of Industrial Toxicology. 2nd ed. John Wiley & Sons, 605 Third Ave., New York, N.Y. 10016, 1959. Out of print.

Many others are listed in the pharmacy college library lists.

For information on determination of poisons in the body, E. G. C. Clarke's *Isolation and Identification of Drugs in Pharmaceuticals, Body Fluids and Postmortem Material* (2 volumes, The Pharmaceutical Press c/o Rittenhouse Book Distributors, 1706 Rittenhouse Sq., Philadelphia, Pa. 19103, 1969, 1975) is a useful source, as is Sunshine's *CRC Manual of Analytical Toxicology* (Chemical Rubber Co., 18901 Cranwood Parkway, Cleveland, Ohio 44128, 1971, $16.00). Alan S. Curry's *Poison Detection in Human Organs* (2nd ed., Charles C Thomas, 301-327 E. Lawrence Ave., Springfield, Ill. 62717, 1969, $13.50) contains detection methods for the fifty-four poisons listed, including such drug groups as barbiturates and monoamine oxidase inhibitors.

Irving Sunshine has also edited the *Handbook of Analytical Toxicology* (Chemical Rubber Co., 18901 Cranwood Parkway, Cleveland, Ohio 44128, 1969, $32.50), which provides an overview of physical and chemical properties, analytical data, and general toxicity of drugs, economic poisons, and industrial chemicals, and standards for air and water analyses.

For antidotes and therapy in general, Poison Information Centers find Dreisbach's *Handbook of Poisoning* (8th ed., Lange Medical Publications, Drawer L, Los Altos, Calif. 94022, 1974. $6.50) about as generally useful as any single text which covers many aspects of acute poisonings. Another source that is widely used and helpful is:

Arena, Jay M.
Poisoning—Toxicology-Sypmtoms-Treatments. 3rd ed.
C. C. Thomas, E. 301-327 Lawrence Ave., Springfield, Ill. 62717, 1974. $43.50.

Finally, those who wish references to further information on the poisoning and its treatment will want to own the following:

Deichmann, William B. and Horace W. Gerarde
Toxicology of Drugs and Chemicals. Academic Press, 111 Fifth Ave., New York, N.Y. 10003, 1969. $35.50. (Paperbound edition, $15.00)

For the research toxicologist, there are the extensive compilations of the National Research Council, *Handbook of Toxicology* (1956-1959; vol. 1, *Acute Toxicities of Solids, Liquids and Gases* to *Laboratory Animals*; vol. 2, *Antibiotics;* vol. 3, *Insecticides;* vol. 4, *Tranquilizers;* vol. 5, *Fungicides*). As implied, these publications deal with toxic levels in laboratory animals and man.

Probably pharmacists in general are more likely to be concerned with adverse effects of drugs and their interactions with other drugs, laboratory tests, or environmental factors, than with a comprehensive poison information collection. As we have already indicated, the drug handbooks contain a good deal of information on side effects and adverse reactions.

To keep up further, one can use the abstract bulletin, *ClinAlert*, the triennial review volume, L. Meyler and A. Herxheimer's *Side Effects of Drugs: A Survey of Unwanted Effects of Drugs Reported in 1968-1971*, Volume 7, Humanities Press (Excerpta Medica, 450 Park Ave. S., New York, N.Y. 10016, 1972, $53.00), and L. Meyler's *Drug-induced Diseases* (Volume 4, American Elsevier Publishing Co., 52 Vanderbilt Ave., New York, N.Y. 10017, 1973, $54.00). The monograph most generally recognized is Robert H. Moser's *Diseases of Medical Progress: A Study of Iatrogenic Disease* (3rd ed., Charles C Thomas, 301-327 E. Lawrence Ave., Springfield, Ill. 62703, 1969, $39.50).

The National Library of Medicine's quarterly *Toxicity Bibliography* provides the titles of journal articles which discuss adverse effects, poisoning, or general chronic or acute toxicity of drugs and chemicals.

There are a great many handbooks on drug interactions. Recent studies[1,2] indicate that the best currently available has been that by Philip D. Hansten, *Drug Interactions* (2nd ed., Lea and Febiger, Washington Square, Philadelphia, Pa. 19106, 1973, $9.50). A major, comprehensive text containing monographs on interactions appeared in June 1973:

American Pharmaceutical Association
Evaluations of Drug Interactions—1973. Prepared by the American Pharmaceutical Association with the cooperation and assistance of the American Dental Association, the American Medical Association, the American Society of Hospital Pharmacists, the Food and Drug Administration, the National Library of Medicine. American Pharmaceutical Association, 2215 Constitution Ave., N.W., Washington, D.C. 20037, 1973. $10.00. *1974 Supplement,* $2.00.

Also recently issued is *Drug Interactions — An Annotated Bibliog-

raphy with Selected Excerpts, 1967-1970, Volume 1 and *1970-1971,* Volume 2, prepared for the National Library of Medicine by Paul deHaen, Government Printing Office, Washington, D.C. 20402. Volume 1: HE 20.3614:D84/967-970/V. 1, S/N 1752-0139, $27.05; Volume 2: HE 20.3614:D84/970-71/V. 2, S/N 1752-00157, $17.70). Mr. deHaen is continuing the publication with his bimonthly *Drug Interactions,* volume 1, 1972, priced at $400.00 a year.

Another important bibliographic series is *Drug Interactions-1* and *Drug Interactions-2,* which together cover a three-year collection of abstracts from *International Pharmaceutical Abstracts.*

Drug Abuse Materials

There has been a flood of publication about drug abuse. All pharmacists will want to provide scientific information about drugs of abuse when asked. For this purpose books on drug abuse will not be as useful as those just mentioned concerning the pharmacology and toxicology of all drugs. However, if the pharmacist wishes more popular materials on illegal drug use, several suggestions can be made.

Many public libraries have recent books on the drug culture in their collections, and some also issue bibliographies listing the relevant book and periodical material they possess. Useful general and specific bibliographies are available from the National Clearinghouse for Drug Abuse Information program (5600 Fishers Lane, Rockville, Md. 20852). This Center also has a computer data base from which it will list reports on specific subjects.

The National Commission on Marihuana and Drug Abuse has issued a complex of reports:

Marihuana: A Signal of Misunderstanding, First Report . . . U.S. Government Printing Office, Washington, D.C. 20402, 1972. Y 3.M 33/2:2M33, S/N 5266-00001, $1.90.

Appendix, Marihuana: A Signal of Misunderstanding, The Technical Papers of the First Report . . . U.S. Government Printing Office, Washington, D.C. 20402, 1972. Y 3.M 33/2:2 M 33/App./V. 1,2, S/N 5266-00002, $12.00 per two-volume set.

Drug Use in America: Problem in Perspective, Second Report

... U.S. Government Printing Office, Washington, D.C. 20402, 1973. Y 3.M 33/2:1/973, S/N 5266-00003, $3.30.

Appendix, Drug Use in America: Problems in Perspective. The Technical Papers of the Second Report ... Volume I: *Patterns and Consequences of Drug Use;* Volume II: *Social Responses to Drug Use;* Volume III: *The Legal System and Drug Control;* and Volume IV: *Treatment and Rehabilitation.* U.S. Government Printing Office, Washington, D.C. 20402, 1973. Y 3.M 33/2:1/973/App/V. 1-4, S/N 5266-00004-7, $11.85, $6.15, $7.40, and $7.45.

In addition, three recent books which have been highly recommended by colleagues are:

Bourne, Peter G., editor
A Treatment Manual for Acute Drug Abuse Emergencies. National Clearinghouse for Drug Abuse Information, National Institute on Drug Abuse, 5600 Fishers Lane, Rockville, Md. 20852, 1974. Available from U.S. Government Printing Office, Washington, D.C. 20402, S/N 1724-00303, $2.15.

Musto, David F.
The American Disease. Origins of Narcotic Control. Yale University Press, 92-A Yale Station, New Haven, Conn. 06520, 1973. $10.95.

World Health Organization. Expert Committee on Drug Dependence.
Twentieth Report. (Technical Report Series #551.) World Health Organization, c/o Q Corporation, 49 Sheridan Avenue, Albany, N.Y. 12210, 1974. $2.80.

For films on drug abuse, one may turn to:

Weber, David O., editor
99+ Films on Drugs. Educational Film Library Association, 17 W. Sixtieth St., New York, N.Y. 10023, 1970. $3.00.

National Coordinating Council on Drug Education
Drug Abuse Films. 3rd ed. (Evaluative report on over 220 films and audiovisuals.) National Coordinating Council on Drug Education, Suite 212, 1211 Connecticut Ave., N.W., Washington, D.C. 20036, 1974. $5.00.

Books on Medicine

Nemec's reference shelf contains a minimum of books in medicine:

Dorland's Illustrated Medical Dictionary. 25th ed. W. B. Saunders Co., W. Washington Sq., Philadelphia, Pa. 19105, 1974. $21.50.

or

Blakiston's New Gould Medical Dictionary. 3rd ed. McGraw-Hill Book Co., 1221 Ave. of the Americas, New York, N.Y. 10020, 1972. $8.75.

or

Stedman, Thomas L.
Stedman's Medical Dictionary. 22nd ed. Williams & Wilkins Co., 428 E. Preston St., Baltimore, Md. 21202, 1972. $18.50.

Brobeck, John R., editor
Best & Taylor's Physiological Basis of Medical Practice. 9th ed. Williams & Wilkins Co., 428 E. Preston St., Baltimore, Md. 21202, 1973. $24.50.

To this group can be added inexpensive, ready reference handbooks, such as the following:

Krupp, Marcus A. and Milton J. Chatton, editors
Current Medical Diagnosis and Treatment. Rev. ed. Lange Medical Publications, Drawer L, Los Altos, Calif. 94022, 1974. $12.00.

Washington University Department of Medicine
Manual of Medical Therapeutics. 20th ed. Edited by Michael G. Rosenfeld. Little, Brown and Co., 34 Beacon St., Boston, Mass. 02106, 1971. $7.50.

Chatton, Milton J.
Handbook of Medical Treatment. 14th ed. Lange Medical Publications, Drawer L, Los Altos, Calif. 94022, 1974. $7.50.

Krupp, Marcus A., Norman J. Sweet, Ernst Jawetz, Edward G. Biglieri and Robert Roe

Physician's Handbook. 17th ed. (Over half on diagnosis and diagnostic tests) Lange Medical Publications, Drawer L, Los Altos, Calif. 94022, 1973. $6.50.

If the pharmacist has special clinical interests, he will want other books. A good place to find a recognized text in a specialty is to look at core lists for libraries such as the Stearns and Ratcliff, "An Integrated Health-Science Core Library for Physicians, Nurses and Allied Health Practitioners," or the Brandon "Selected List of Books and Journals for the Small Medical Library" (See Table 5). In some cases, the pharmacist may find that a text different from the one generally recognized suits his needs, but he can scarcely go wrong in specialties of possible interest with those listed below:

INTERNAL MEDICINE   Beeson, Paul B. and W. McDermott, editors
Cecil-Loeb Textbook of Medicine. 13th ed. W. B. Saunders Co., W. Washington Sq., Philadelphia, Pa. 19105, 1971. Single vol., $26.00; 2 vols., $30.00.

Wintrobe, Maxwell M., R. D. Adams, I. L. Bennett, E. Braunwald, K. Isselbacher, R. Petersdorf and G. W. Thorne, editors
Harrison's Principles of Internal Medicine. 7th ed. McGraw-Hill Book Co., 1221 Ave. of the Americas, New York, N.Y. 10020, 1974. 2 vols. $35.00.

PEDIATRICS   Vaughn, Victor C. and R. James McKay, editors
Nelson Textbook of Pediatrics. 10th ed. W. B. Saunders Co., W. Washington Sq., Philadelphia, Pa. 19105, 1975. $32.75

Shirkey, Harry C., editor
Pediatric Therapy. 4th ed. C. V. Mosby Co., 11830 Westline Dr., St. Louis, Mo. 63141, 1972. $34.50.

LIVER DISEASE   Sherlock, Sheila
Diseases of the Liver and Biliary System. 5th ed. F. A. Davis Co., 1915 Arch St., Philadelphia, Pa. 19103, 1975. Price not set.

KIDNEY DISEASE	Strauss, Maurice B. and Louis G. Welt *Diseases of the Kidney.* 2nd ed. Little, Brown and Co., 34 Beacon St., Boston, Mass. 02106, 1971. 2 vols. $50.00.
NEUROLOGY	Merritt, H. Houston *Textbook of Neurology.* 5th ed. Lea and Febiger, Washington Sq., Philadelphia, Pa. 19106, 1973. $18.50.
ENDOCRINOLOGY	Williams, Robert H., editor *Textbook of Endocrinology.* 5th ed. W. B. Saunders Co., W. Washington Sq., Philadelphia, Pa. 19105, 1974. $28.00.
MICROBIOLOGY	Davis, Bernard D., Renato Dulbecco, Herman N. Eisen and Harold S. Ginsberg *Microbiology,* 2nd ed., Harper & Row, Scranton, Pa. 18512, 1973. $27.50.
OPHTHALMOLOGY	Newell, Frank W. *Ophthalmology: Principles and Concepts.* 3rd ed. C. V. Mosby Co., 11830 Westline Dr., St. Louis, Mo. 63141, 1974. $19.50.

Books on Chemistry

The bibliographies by Jackson and Zachert and Thomasson (Table 5) are excellent sources for almost any specific works on inorganic, organic, and medicinal chemistry and on biochemistry.

Physicians' lists (Inke, Brandon, and Stearns, Table 5) seem to agree on:

White, Abraham
Principles of Biochemistry. 5th ed. McGraw-Hill Book Co., 1221 Ave. of the Americas, New York, N.Y. 10020, 1973. $19.95.

I cannot find fault with Nemec's selections in medicinal chemistry:

Burger, Alfred
Medicinal Chemistry. 3rd ed. John Wiley & Sons, 605 Third

Ave., New York, N.Y. 10016, 1970. Parts 1 and 2, $42.50 each.

or

Wilson, Charles Owens, Ole Gisvold and Robert F. Doerge
Textbook of Organic Medicinal and Pharmaceutical Chemistry. 6th ed. J. B. Lippincott Co., E. Washington Sq., Philadelphia, Pa. 19105, 1971. $24.00.

For pharmacists, the choices in organic and inorganic chemistry are probably not so critical. They will find adequate information in the sources already cited, plus *Chemical Publications* or another guide to the chemical literature. Pasztor and Hopkins is also very comprehensive in its chemistry listing (See Table 5).

There remains one important area — clinical chemistry — which will concern the pharmacist because of possible drug-induced irregularities in test results. Brandon lists a number of books in this field, from which I have selected the following:

Davidsohn, Israel and John Bernard Henry, editors
Todd-Sandford Clinical Diagnosis by Laboratory Methods. 15th ed. W. B. Saunders Co., W. Washington Sq., Philadelphia, Pa. 19105, 1974. $28.00.

Widmann, Frances K.
Goodale's Clinical Interpretation of Laboratory Tests. 7th ed. F. A. Davis Co., 1915 Arch St., Philadelphia, Pa. 19103, 1973. $12.95.

Levinson, Samuel Azor and Robert P. MacFate
Clinical Laboratory Diagnosis. 7th ed. Lea and Febiger, Washington Sq., Philadelphia, Pa. 19106, 1969. $28.50.

Clinical chemists will also need the following:
Young, D. S., L. C. Postaner and Val Gibberman
"Effects of Drugs on Clinical Laboratory Tests." *Clinical Chemistry* 21: ID-432D, Apr. 1975. Available separately from American Association of Clinical Chemists, 1725 K St., N.W., Washington, DC 20006. $10.00

Constantino, Norma V. and Hugh F. Kabat
"Drug-induced Modifications of Laboratory Test Values — Revised 1973." *American Journal of Hospital Pharmacy* 30: 24-71, Jan. 1973. Sold separately for $2.00.

References

1. Bell, J. Edward. "A Comparative Evaluation of Drug Interaction Publications." *American Journal of Hospital Pharmacy* 18:938-944, Dec. 1971.

2. Sewell, Winifred. "Drug Interactions as a Communications Problem." *Drug Information Journal* 6:6-11, Jan.-June 1972.

CHAPTER 9

OTHER PRIMARY SOURCES

Manufacturers' Literature

Some printed materials used by pharmacists do not fall into the categories of books, journals, handbooks and secondary sources. Pre-eminent among them is the body of manufacturers' literature. This can be divided into many classes from simple reminders on specific drugs through package inserts to rather comprehensive brochures or extensive bibliographies. In addition, some companies issue house organs directed to the pharmacist or the physician or both. Available free of charge, they include such examples as the following:

Pharmacy News — Smith Kline & French Laboratories
Hospital Pharmacy (The "White Sheet") — Philips Roxane Laboratories, Inc.
Hospital Pharmacy News — Eli Lilly & Company
Hypertension Bulletin (Hospital Tribune) — Ciba Pharmaceutical Company
Tile and Till — Eli Lilly & Company
Ciba-Geigy Journal — Ciba Corporation, Basel, Switzerland
Triangle, Journal of Medical Science — Sandoz-Wander, Inc., Basel, Switzerland

Though practically every company issued a house organ ten or twenty years ago,[1] the practice has pretty much died out now.

Instead, manufacturers have supported such newspaper-type publications as *Medical Tribune, Medical World News,* and *Hospital Tribune,* which are widely distributed to physicians and other health professionals and which carry extensive advertising.

Of special interest is *The Lilly Digest, A Survey of Community Pharmacy Operations,* which is distributed annually and has extensive tables on sales, income, expenses, and other aspects of the business operation of a pharmacy.

If a company's representative visits you regularly, ask him for library bibliographies on a product in which you are interested. Most pharmaceutical libraries maintain extensive product reference lists, which tend to have more complete information than you could obtain in a search of the literature. For practical reasons, they are not always available outside the company.

If you receive such a bibliography explore its scope and limitations. Depending on the guidelines in its preparation, such a list may contain every single mention of a manufacturer's product, however insignificant. This would diminish its usefulness for substantive information unless it provided abstracts or annotations. On the other hand, if the compilation is for internal use by scientific staff, it may cover significant papers on both the company product and competitive ones. If you are going to rely on such bibliographies, you should check them for inclusion of papers you have found in a different way.

Sometimes companies put out bibliographies not directly related to marketed products, such as the five volumes on *Cyclic AMP* (1957-1969, 1970, 1971, 1972, and 1973) issued by E. R. Squibb & Sons.

You may want to maintain a file of package inserts for ready access to what the FDA has agreed the manufacturer may say about his product. (Remember that essentially the same information is in *Physicians' Desk Reference,* though not for all products.) You will find that the information given on the package insert is neither complete nor necessarily balanced.

There has been a great deal written on the influence on the physician of the manufacturer's literature — from package insert through direct mail advertising to advertising in journals.[2-5] In developing his own attitude toward this literature, the pharmacist should remember:

1. Much information can be obtained from the manufacturer.

2. The physician and dentist see the manufacturer's literature. The pharmacist will need to see it too in order to anticipate the prescriber's behavior, as well as to discuss the drug with him.

3. The primary motive of the manufacturer has to be to sell his products. One should ask if there is any evident bias or if there may be other published information on the product which the manufacturer is not distributing.

4. The pharmacist should have alternative sources of information so that he can decide on their validity himself, and avoid dependence on any channel, including the manufacturer.

A good list of all sorts of substantive publications of pharmaceutical companies, as well as other "free or inexpensive industrial or institutional pamphlet material of an informative nature," was *COPNIP List*, issued by the Pharmaceutical Division of the Special Libraries Association. (Recently it was edited by Mrs. Theodora Andrews and distributed for $3.00 annually by Alberta D. Berton, College of Physicians of Philadelphia, 19 S. 22nd St., Philadelphia, Pa. 19103.) It was discontinued in 1975.

Patents

Another type of special publication which pharmacists should understand is patents. Perhaps the most important fact for the average pharmacist to know is that patents contain original information on product formulations that may not be found anywhere else in the literature — for a patent is a part of the literature, even though it may not be kept in most medical libraries.

American patents can be granted to individuals when they have discovered a new chemical substance or a new process for making an old chemical substance. Rarely, a patent will be issued for a new use for an old substance, such as the method of treating tuberculosis with isoniazid.[6] Hence there may be more than one patent related to a single product.

There are usually two parts to a patent, disclosures and claims. The disclosure describes what has been discovered, and may discuss why it is important. The claim tells what the inventor registers as his legal right under the patent.

A United States patent grants to an individual or individuals exclusive rights for seventeen years to manufacture the products or use the processes claimed in the patent. During that time, others may not use any procedure or make any product claimed in the patent without permission (licensing). While the U.S. Patent Office grants patents only to individuals, in practice a research scientist usually signs an agreement with his employer that anything discovered while he is working for the company will belong to it. Because the company is named in the patent as an assignee, we often speak of it as receiving the patent. In some countries, the industrial organization actually does obtain the patent.

A patent does not establish the efficacy or safety of a drug. The Food and Drug Administration regulates those aspects of the product through its approval for marketing.

It is useful to know the original patent number and date if one is making a literature search on a drug, since this will enable one to predict when toxicity and animal studies may have been published. The date of issuance is determined by the date of the *Official Gazette of the U.S. Patent Office* in which the patent is announced. The patent also has an application date, which facilitates relating it to its equivalents throughout the world, since the applications are usually filed in a number of countries at the same time. A patent may require two or three years for processing. Although formerly it was possible for a drug to be marketed before the patent had been issued, today the date of issuance is likely to precede the date of an approved New Drug Application, often by years.

There is an extensive discussion of patent literature and its searching in Mellon's *Chemical Publications* (See Table 5).

Copies of American patents and some foreign ones may be purchased directly from the U.S. Patent Office if they are not available in a local industrial or public library. To find the current method of obtaining copies from the Patent Office, check the first January issue of *Chemical Abstracts* under "Procurement of Patents" in the section on "Suggestions for Procurement of Copies of Original Documents Abstracted in Chemical Abstracts."

Government Documents

Many government documents are discussed as periodicals, monographs, or abstracting and indexing services in other parts of this book. They are mentioned here separately as well because the pharmacist may be unaware of a great many of possible interest. Those of the U.S. Government come from the legislative, executive, and judicial branches and are sometimes difficult to locate.

One bibliography is *Drugstores* by Joseph D. McEvilla (U.S. Government Printing Office, Washington, D.C. 20402, April 1970). It is published by the Small Business Administration and is available free from that source in Washington or its field offices. Both government and nongovernment publications are listed and a number of other sources of information on government publications are included.

The Superintendent of Documents (U.S. Government Printing Office (GPO), Washington, D.C. 20402) is the major source of publications, most of which are free or very inexpensive in relation to their value. If you wish to keep up with major new publications of general interest, there is a monthly *Selected Government Publications*, which will be sent regularly if you request it from the GPO. There are also *Price Lists* in special areas, such as *Government Periodicals and Subscription Services (Price List 36)*, or *Tariff and Taxation (Price List 37)*, or *Diseases and Physical Conditions, Alcoholism, Dentistry, Drugs and Narcotics Addiction, Smoking, and Vital and Health Statistics (Price List 51A)*. More elaborate bibliographic sources of government publications are maintained in most large university and public libraries.

The kinds of material which can be obtained free from Congress are also very helpful. If you have seen in the news that there is a Congressional investigation of particular interest, you may obtain the Committee hearings by writing to the Chairman of the Committee. Probably your own Congressman would be glad to forward your request to the appropriate person. These Hearings frequently are a major source of kinds of information not readily obtained elsewhere. For instance, an extensive compilation of advertising expenditures and sales revenues for a variety of nonproprietary drugs is found in the testimony of Dr. Michael Mann (Director, Bureau of Economics, Federal Trade Commission) in the Hearings before the Subcommittee on Monopoly of the Select Committee on Small Business.[7]

In recent years, the "report literature" has become very extensive. During and following World War II, much scientific and technical investigation has been done by industry and universities

OTHER PRIMARY SOURCES 89

under government contracts. Reports of the work may or may not have appeared in the regular primary literature — journals or textbooks. In the technical or engineering field, particularly, many are available only from the government. The major source of such technical reports is the National Technical Information Service (NTIS) (The U.S. Department of Commerce, 5285 Port Royal Road, Springfield, Virginia 22151).

Recently this organization has become a depository for other government documents that are not likely to be so widely distributed as publications of the Superintendent of Documents (GPO). As an example, NTIS publishes the special indexing and searching tools used in MEDLINE — the National Library of Medicine's computerized, on-line, bibliographic searching system discussed in Chapters 13 and 16. Another example is the *Desktop Analysis Tool for the Common Data Base*, which is a listing of the chemical names, all synonyms, and registry numbers for about 30,000 compounds — drugs, pesticides, colors, cosmetics, etc. — prepared by Chemical Abstracts Service for several government agencies. This is available from NTIS for $100.00. Most of the materials can be purchased from NTIS either as regular "hard copy" or in microfiche (See Chapter 18).

To tell what materials are distributed by NTIS, one can consult the following:

Government Research Announcements (GRA; formerly *U.S. Government Research and Development Reports).* Semimonthly abstracts of 60,000 reports annually in all fields.

Government Research Index (GRI; formerly *U.S. Government Research and Development Reports Index).* Concurrent index to *GRA* by subject, personal and corporate authors, and by government contract and order numbers.

Government Reports Technical Announcements (GRTA; formerly *Clearinghouse Announcements in Science and Technology).* Published semimonthly in separate but highly defined fields such as Biological and Medical Sciences; Biotechnology and Medical Engineering; Chemistry. It will be replaced gradually by *Weekly Government Abstracts* in similar fields.

If you are not sure whether NTIS has publications on your question, you can call or write them to ask for a search on their computerized data base.

If one cannot find information in any publication, one can call on the National Referral Center of the Science and Technology Division within the Library of Congress. This center is different from the NTIS or the GPO in that it will refer one to people or organizations who can answer questions rather than to publications. One of its major means of accomplishing this function is to publish directories of governmental and nongovernmental sources of information, such as:

> A *Directory of Information Resources in the United States. General Toxicology.* Compiled . . . for the Toxicology Information Program, National Library of Medicine. June 1969.

> A *Directory of Information Resources in the United States. Biological Sciences.* 1972.

Some of the professional pharmacy journals — *American Journal of Hospital Pharmacy* and *American Journal of Pharmaceutical Education* — list government publications of interest to their readers. Following these lists is the easiest way for the pharmacist to be aware of some of the wealth of information available from the government.

Theses and Research Studies

A kind of information that will not be very often used by the pharmacist is the thesis. Most doctoral dissertations in the biological and physical sciences are condensed and appear in the journal literature. Masters' theses also will appear there if they are considered to be worth it. If one has occasion to find an original thesis, it will usually be available on microfilm. Libraries have extensive lists of doctoral dissertations in the current *Dissertation Abstracts* and its *Dissertation Abstracts International Retrospective Index.*

Perhaps more pertinent to pharmacists' current interests is the "Index of Current Studies in Hospital Pharmacy" which appears irregularly in the *American Journal of Hospital Pharmacy.*

The Smithsonian Science Information Exchange, Inc. (1730 M Street, N.W., Washington, D.C. 20036) provides abstracts of research in progress, "Notices of Research Projects," either in response to a specific request or through Special Interest Packages on topics of current interest announced in the *SSIE Science Newsletter*. Research projects supported by the National Institutes of Health are described in its *Research Grants Index*.

Another kind of information source not in regular printed form — audiovisuals — is discussed in Chapter 18.

References

1. Maurice, Jewell. "The Development, Criteria for Selection and Uses of House Organs." *Bulletin of the Medical Library Association* 40:341-347 Oct. 1952.

2. McLaughlin, Curtis P., and Roy Penchansky. "Diffusion of Innovation in Medicine: a Problem of Continuing Medical Education." *Journal of Medical Education* 40:437-447, May 1965.

3. Coleman, James S., Elihu Katz and Herbert Menzel. *Medical Innovation, a Diffusion Study*. Bobbs-Merrill, Indianapolis, 1966. P. 53.

4. Ben Gaffin and Associates. *Attitudes of U.S. Physicians Toward the American Pharmaceutical Industry*. American Medical Association, Chicago, 1959. Through reference 3.

5. Sherrington, Andrew M. "An Annotated Bibliography of Studies on the Flow of Medical Information to Practitioners." *Methods of Information in Medicine* 4:45-57, Jan. 1965.

6. Forman, Howard I., editor. *The Law of Chemical, Metallurgical and Pharmaceutical Patents*. Central Book Co., Inc., New York, 1967. P. 70.

7. U.S. Senate, Ninety-second Congress, First Session. *Hearings before the Subcommittee on Monopoly of the Select Committee on Small Business*. (Gaylord Nelson, Chairman). "Advertising of Proprietary Medicines. Effect of Promotion and Advertising of Over-the-Counter Drugs on Competition, Small Business, and the Health and Welfare of the Public. Part 1. May 25, 26; June 15 and 17, 1971. Introduction; Analgesics." U.S. Government Printing Office, Washington, D.C. 20402, 1971. $1.75, Stock Number 5270-1200.

CHAPTER 10

DIRECTORIES, DICTIONARIES, EQUIPMENT CATALOGS, AND OTHER REFERENCE SOURCES

One cannot predict all the pharmacist's needs for factual data — an address, the meaning of a word, some kind of statistics — that would be found in what librarians call "ready reference sources." It is easier for the author and reader to leave these sources to the individual reference librarian at the time of the specific question. The following discussion of a few sources is limited to strict pharmacy or recognizable immediate needs of the pharmacist. Remember that dictionaries in chemistry or medicine may sometimes be more useful than a pharmaceutical dictionary, even for a pharmacy question.

A good source of all sorts of miscellaneous facts and statistics about drugs is the *Final Report. Summary of Major Findings* of the Task Force on Prescription Drugs (Office of the Secretary, U.S. Department of Health, Education and Welfare, 1969. Out of print.) Other statistics will be found largely in journals — such periodic studies as that of store sales by departments in *American Druggist* and the chain drug industry annual report which appears in *Chain Store Age, Drug Executives Edition*, in the late spring. A list of statistical sources for pharmacists has been published by Nelson Weindling.[1]

Directories of manufacturers are found in many of the drug handbooks as indicated in the first section. To find personnel in key positions in pharmaceutical firms, as well as general information on the company, one may use *Executive Directory of the U.S.*

Pharmaceutical Industry, edited by K. R. Kern (Chemical Economic Services, Princeton, 1972. $35.00). Pharmacies currently licensed can be found in the National Association of Boards of Pharmacy *Directory of Licensed Pharmacies* (77 W. Washington, Chicago, Ill. 60602), updated monthly. Pharmacists may also be familiar with *The Hayes Druggists' Directory and Commercial Reference Book* (Edward N. Hayes, Santa Ana, Calif., biennial) which gives gross financial and credit information.

Equipment directories — like manufacturers' drug price lists — will probably come to those who need them automatically, through salesmen or direct mail from the manufacturers. Pharmacists are concerned with many different kinds of equipment beyond those directly involving medicaments. A recent list of "Manufacturers of Hospital Pharmacy Equipment and Supplies" should also be of interest to other pharmacists.[2] The categories of material contained in it are: Administrative Furnishings and Filing Equipment and Supplies; Communication Equipment; Computer Systems; Equipment and Supplies for Medications and Materials Handling; Equipment and Supplies for Packaging Oral Solids, Oral Liquids, Injectables and Miscellaneous Drug Products; Equipment and Supplies for Printing and Labeling; Microfilm Readers, Printers and Supplies; Pharmacy and Medical Records Forms; Storage Facilities and Refrigerators; and Miscellaneous Equipment and Supplies.

Some valuable directory information is found in journals. Examples are the list of pharmacy schools and their deans which appears each year as "Institutions Holding Membership in the American Association of Colleges of Pharmacy" in the *American Journal of Pharmaceutical Education,* or the periodic lists of officers of state pharmaceutical associations which is from time to time in the feature, "Pharmacy — Today and Tomorrow" in the *Journal of the American Pharmaceutical Association.* Until recently a great deal of directory and other information about hospitals — for instance, total payroll figures for each — could be obtained in Part 2 of the August 1 issue of *Hospitals.* Now that publication has been separated into the *AHA Guide to the Health Care Field* (American Hospital Association, 840 N. Lake Shore Drive, Chicago, Ill. 60611, 1973).

There is no good pharmaceutical dictionary in English, but that by Curt Hunnius in German (*Pharmazeutisches Wörterbuch,* 5th edition. W. DeGruyter, Berlin, 1974) is excellent. Interesting-

ly, there are three polyglot dictionaries all issued at about the same time ten years ago. Since each covers different languages and different words, all should ideally be available. They are:
English, French, German Italian, Latin:

> Graa, Albert. *Vocabularium Pharmaceuticum, in vier Sprachen, mit einem Index der lateinischen Abkurzungen für die Rezeptur.* 2nd edition. Helbing & Lichtenhahn, Basel, Switzerland, 1964.

English, French, German, Italian, Spanish, Greek, Russian:

> Steinbichler, Evaline
> *Steinbichler's Lexikon für die Apothekenpraxis in sieben Sprachen, mit fünf selbabstandigen Alphabeten und einer pharmazeutischen Phraseologie.* Govi-Verlag, Frankfurt/Main, Germany, 1963.

English, French, German, Italian, Spanish — for pharmaceutical technology:

> *Elsevier's Dictionary of Pharmaceutical Science and Techniques, in Five Languages.* Volume 1. *Pharmaceutical Technology.* Elsevier Publishing Co., New York, 1968.

Sources of general facts and figures in pharmacy and medicine are:

> Pharmaceutical Society of Great Britain
> *Pharmaceutical Handbook, incorporating the Pharmaceutical Pocket Book,* edited by R. G. Todd. 18th ed. Pharmaceutical Press, c/o Rittenhouse Book Distributors, 1706 Rittenhouse Sq., Philadelphia, Pa. 19103, 1970. $8.50. (Point of view is primarily British and a great deal of material is included on preparation and sterilization of medicines.)

> Documenta Geigy
> *Scientific Tables,* edited by K. Diem and C. Lentner. 7th ed. Ciba-Geigy, Ltd., Basel, Switzerland, 1970. (Distributed by Geigy Pharmaceuticals, Div. of Ciba-Geigy Corp., Ardsley, N.Y. 10502.) This combines in one volume information one would expect to find in several: biological data and normal clinical laboratory values along with physical, chemical, and mathematical tables.)

A reference manual in hospital pharmacy intended primarily as a guide to standards is the American Hospital Association's *Reference Manual on Hospital Pharmacy* (840 N. Lake Shore Drive, Chicago, Ill. 60611, 1970. $5.25.)

References

1. Weindling, Nelson. "Statistical Sources for Pharmacists." *Journal of the American Pharmaceutical Association* NS14:26-30, 40, Jan. 1974.
2. Northern, Robert E. and Thomas R. Brown. "Manufacturers of Hospital Pharmacy Equipment and Supplies." *American Journal of Hospital Pharmacy* 30:1038-1049, Nov. 1973. A separate of the listing is being sold by the American Society of Hospital Pharmacists (4630 Montgomery Ave., Washington, D.C. 20014) for $0.75.

CHAPTER *11*

PART 3

GOING BEYOND ONE'S OWN COLLECTION

It is important to have a first-rate collection at hand because many of the questions a pharmacist wishes to answer cannot wait for a half-hour or hour while he makes a phone call, let alone a half-day or more to go to a library or other source of in-depth information. Yet the match between the thousands of papers which may have some bearing on a single question and the few that a pharmacist can keep at hand is so poor that he will reach a limit in the questions he can answer with his own collection. Hopefully, he will build his collection so that he can answer 90 percent of his needs locally. We should like to turn now to the other 10 percent that will require assistance from a library or drug information center of some kind. Although the pharmacist often can get an answer by means of a phone call, he will find it helpful to have some familiarity with the resources of the librarian or drug information specialist at the other end of the wire. In addition, while he is getting his education, and continuing to expand it over the years, he will need to use libraries for his own in-depth research. This section is therefore being written as though the pharmacist will be doing all his own searching, even though the ideal situation will be for much of it to be done for him.

Many of the useful sources of information to which the pharmacist will turn will not involve the literature directly. One such source, the manufacturer, has been discussed in Chapter 9.

Another — and perhaps the most frequently used — is the exchange of information with colleagues. However, it is the purpose of this book to concentrate on the help the pharmacist can get from the literature, and he will probably turn first to the library when he goes beyond his own collection.

We will discuss first the library in general, then the abstracts, indexes, and other reference sources where he may find help, and finally the resources the library may turn to when a question cannot be answered locally.

The Library

The library is, of course, more than a collection of books. It includes staff members whose function is to assist and guide their "clientele" in finding what is wanted. And it includes an organization, much like that in a retail store, for collecting and organizing materials so that they can be found by the library user, the consumer. In a well equipped, fully staffed library, this organization also provides for culling outdated books from the shelf much as outdated produce is removed from the supermarket. Unfortunately, many libraries have not been adequately staffed to carry out all these functions effectively.

As a librarian who has used the library for personal research all her life, I may be more critical than the average consumer. My frustrations do not always derive from major policies involving the organization of the collection or the selection and purchasing of books for it. They arise, instead, from such minor matters as the change of shelf location of a favorite book because the collection has been shifted; the unavailability of needed items because they are on loan, at the bindery, waiting to be shelved, or simply "lost"; or the complexities of differing loan policies for different materials. I cannot offer any simple solutions to these problems, only commiseration and the recommendation that you let the library staff know specifically about each problem rather than as a general expression of dissatisfaction. In a situation in which rules have to be established to satisfy many different and often conflicting needs, the problems which are expressed most vocally and most succinctly will tend to get most attention.

Perhaps a few words about the general organization of the library will help to take some of the mystery from it, and thus to reduce the number of problems. For more details one should turn to local library guides.

The Collection

Traditionally, the vast bulk of the library will be divided into two sections: the books, and the periodicals or serials. Practices differ with respect to the handling of annuals and other periodic publications which fall between the traditional journal, published quarterly, monthly, or more frequently, and the traditional book, published once and reissued as a complete new edition if there is sufficient demand. In some libraries everything published annually or less frequently is part of the book collection; in others everything published annually or more frequently is part of the journal collection. Some libraries list all serial titles along with book titles in their general card catalog, while others have two quite separate and independent files, a card catalog for books, and a title and holdings file for serials. It takes relatively little time to introduce oneself to the practices of a particular library, but failure to do so can be catastrophic. An experienced library user, coming to an unfamiliar library, assumed it did not have *California Medicine* because he did not find it in the card catalog, yet it was listed in the serials file of the library, with holdings complete from 1924!

Three smaller parts of the collection may not present problems. Most university undergraduates are familiar with the reserve reading room in which most health science school libraries keep books assigned in particular courses. A book you are looking for may be held there for others, even though it has not been assigned in any of your courses. Anyone who has used a library has probably encountered the reference collection — those biographical and organizational directories, encyclopedias, encyclopedic texts, handbooks, and other works frequently used for reference, which are hence not to be taken from the library. Finally, some libraries have a documents collection — publications of various governmental organizations, state, local, national, and international (such as the World Health Organization). In many libraries, all documents are treated like any other books and serials, but in others, some documents are separated so that they need not be fully cataloged. Instead, indexes published by the issuing agencies serve as a guide to them. In thorough research, the documents collection should be checked in any library which has one.

A few libraries will have some subject or memorial collections housed separately. Be sure to notice these in local library guides or during orientation sessions to see if they are potentially useful. There may also be a history reading room, groups of theses accepted in local schools, or publications by faculty, etc. Unless he is a history buff, the pharmacist is not likely to find these collections significant in his search of the literature.

Whether there is a separate pharmacy school library or the pharmacy students use a health science library intended for other health science students as well, there will be formal or informal departmental libraries in the pharmacy school — collections primarily for the use of faculty and graduate students. If the beginning student is encouraged to use them, he should remember to be familiar also with the broader resources of the general library. On the other hand, if a crucial book or periodical is missing from the general library, he should remember to check these departmental collections.

Organization of the Collection

There are many different possible classification schemes, including those created expressly for an individual library. The three systems that the user of a pharmacy-oriented library in America is most likely to encounter are: National Library of Medicine, Library of Congress, and Dewey Decimal. Since one can find the classification number from the card catalog, one's concern with the classification itself can be secondary. For those who are interested, the following broad and selective outlines tell where to find some pharmacy-related materials in the three mentioned above:

NATIONAL LIBRARY OF MEDICINE

QS-QZ	Preclinical Sciences
QV	Pharmacology
QV 1-356	General
QV 600-667	Toxicology
QV 701-835	Pharmacy and Pharmaceutics (Note, however, that materials on pharmacy are placed throughout the pharmacology section. Pharmacy as a Profession is included under QV 21, for instance, and Registration of Pharmacists, under QV 29.)
W-WZ	Medicine and Related Subjects (including, for example:)
W	Medical Profession
WA	Public Health

WB	Practice of Medicine
WC	Infectious Diseases
. . . . .	
WE-WL	Diseases by Body System
. . . . .	
WT	Geriatrics. Chronic Disease
WU	Dentistry. Oral Surgery
WV	Otorhinolaryngology
WW	Ophthalmology
WX	Hospitals
WY	Nursing
WZ	History of Medicine

(The National Library of Medicine uses the Library of Congress system for all nonmedical books.)

LIBRARY OF CONGRESS

Q		Science
	QD	Chemistry
	QK	Botany
	QM	Human Anatomy
	QP	Physiology
	QP 903-981	Experimental Pharmacology (with 911 to 981 including chemical substances)
	QR	Bacteriology
R		Medicine
	RA	Public Aspects of Medicine
	RB	Pathology
	. . . . .	
	RM	Therapeutics. Pharmacology
	RM 139	Prescription Writing
	RM 143	Incompatibilities in Prescription
	RM 145	Dose Books
	RM 147-180	Administration of Drugs and Other Therapeutic Agents
	RM 300-666	Drugs and Their Action
	RS	Pharmacy and Materia Medica
	RS 125-151	Formularies, Pharmacopeias, and Dispensatories
	RS 153-441	Materia Medica
	RS 160-167	Pharmacognosy
	RS 402-431	Medical and Pharmaceutical Chemistry

DEWEY DECIMAL

500	Pure Sciences
541-547	Chemistry and Allied Sciences
. . . . .	
600	Technology (Applied Sciences)

610		Medical Sciences
	615	Therapeutics and Pharmacology
	615.1-615.3	Pharmacology and Pharmacy
	615.1	General Pharmacology and Materia Medica
	615.11	Pharmacopeias
	615.12	Dispensatories
	615.13	Formularies
	615.14	Posology. Prescription Writing, Dosage Determination, Incompatibilities
	615.19	Pharmaceutical Chemistry. Manufacture, Preparation, Analysis of Drugs, Medicinals, Biological Products
	615.2-615.3	Specific Groups and Kinds of Pharmaceuticals
	615.4	Practical Pharmacy. Preparing Prescriptions and Dispensing Drugs
	615.5	Therapeutics
	615.6	Methods of Medication
	615.7	Pharmacodynamics. Physiological and Therapeutic Action of Drugs
	615.9	Toxicology. Source, Composition, Physiological Effects, Tests, Antidotes of Poisons
	616	Medicine
	616.1-616.9	Specific Diseases
	617-618	Specialized Medicine
	619	Comparative and Experimental Medicine

Periodicals are sometimes arranged according to the same subject classifications as are books, but in health science libraries they are usually separate and are arranged alphabetically by title. In some libraries, the alphabet is followed strictly (e.g., *Journal of the American Pharmaceutical Association* among the J's), while in others, the journal is alphabetized according to the society which publishes it, if that society forms part of the name (e.g., *Journal of the American Pharmaceutical Association* among the A's).

The Catalog

The card catalog is an indispensable guide to the collection, telling whether the library has a specific book, what books the library possesses on certain topics, and under what call numbers books will be found. All the information — author, title, and subject — may be filed in a single alphabet or the catalog may be divided, usually with authors and titles in one part and subjects in the other.

When working with a catalog in which both titles and subjects appear in a single alphabet, the library user should learn to distinguish between them, because he will not find all available material on a topic until he has checked through all the cards with the corresponding index heading, as well as those for all appropriate subject headings to which he has been referred by cross reference cards under the first topic. The subject frequently appears in red type or all in capital letters, whereas a book title is in black type, or in capital and small letters. A book title is usually longer, more explicit, and also unique.

Though rather elaborate filing rules are used in the card catalog, they affect relatively few cards. If you are looking under a subject or government agency for which there are many entries, you should probably seek assistance from a librarian. Knowledge of whether the following conventions are used in your library will also help:

1. Titles which begin with so-called trivial words are omitted. (e.g., *Textbook of Pharmacology* or *Principles of Pharmacy*) These books will be found under author or subject only.

2. Articles — "*a*," "*an*," "*the*" and their equivalents in foreign languages — are ignored in filing. (*The Pharmacological Basis of Therapeutics* is filed under "Pharmacological.")

3. Abbreviations and numerals are filed as if spelled out. ("St. Louis" is filed between "Safety" and "Sanity." "1969" comes between "Nineham" and "Nippon.")

4. Vowels modified with an umlaut are filed as if followed by an "e." ("Gäre" is filed as if it were "Gaere.")

5. "Mac," "Mc," and "M'" are all filed as if spelled "Mac." ("M'Donald," "McDuffy," and "MacElhaney" appear in that order.)

6. If a single word stands for a person, a place, a subject, and a title word, the cards for the various aspects are filed in the order just listed. ("Paris, Judith" (person) before "Paris, France" (place) before "PARIS" (subject) before "Paris in the Springtime" (title).)

You may notice that the cards in the catalog provide information other than author, title, subject, and call number. Publisher, place, date, and edition number are familiar because they are commonly used in bibliographies. The next information on the card is usually a physical description of the volume — number of pages, illustrative materials, etc. Then there may be a description of special features in the book — extensive bibliographies, or separate sections with different titles or the name of a series to which the volume belongs. Finally, a "main entry" card will list all the terms under which the card is filed in the catalog — topics, title, various authors, etc. Usually the "main entry" card is that for the first author, but when printed cards are used the filing information appears on all of them.

Now that libraries use computers for various functions, it is not unusual to find all or a part of the card catalog in book form. The basic elements and their arrangement remain the same, but copies are available in more than one location.

CHAPTER 12

THE SEARCH

The first step in deciding where to look for information is to make sure you understand what you are looking for. Check all unfamiliar terms in a dictionary. Find a textbook, handbook, or review which discusses your problem in general if you are not sure of its implications.

When you have defined your problem, the next step is to plan how you are going to solve it. I'd like to make a plea for effective use of the pharmacist's time when he goes to the library. Searching efficiency will depend on four actions: advance determination of the level of effort that is required; careful organization of one's work; judicious selection and intelligent use of literature sources; and evaluation of the technique used to assure that the best available information has been found.

Level of Effort

The amount of effort one expends to answer a question always should depend on its purpose. Research toward an advanced degree will require many hours in the library for assurance that everything previously done in the general area of the thesis topic has been reviewed. In a search designed merely to satisfy curiosity, patience may be exhausted after a half-hour of following fruitless leads.

If you are conducting the search for yourself, you can easily determine how far to go, but if the question was asked by someone else, some insight in advance may help you to organize your efforts profitably. If the problem involves a particular patient, the need to get the best and most authoritative information must be balanced against the time remaining before the patient should receive the medication being questioned. The nurse's needs will be satisfied by a more pragmatic answer than the physician's, since the latter must make therapeutic decisions based on sound theory as well as experience.

Sometimes it will be advisable to respond to an immediate need as best you can, later searching thoroughly to fill in your own background and that of your colleagues before a similar question arises again. The danger is that the pharmacist will limit his effort because of ignorance of sources of added information that are both quick and convenient to use. For this reason, it is particularly important that he check later urgent questions which he first answered superficially so that he will be aware of better sources for better answers next time.

Organization of Work

One means of avoiding needless wasted time is keeping good records of each search. These records are of two kinds: sources checked and references found.

Sources checked (see Figure 1) should contain source, date, volume and issue number, kind of index — author, subject, or special — and all the terms used in each index. A grid is very useful, since sources searched can be listed on the horizontal axis and terms used, across the vertical one. University bookstores have notebook paper with evenly spaced horizontal and vertical lines which simplifies this record keeping. If an index refers by numbers to a separate abstract or title section, the numbers can be put in the grid in the course of searching, and the possibly pertinent references reviewed after you have listed them all (See Figure 1).

Keeping this record will permit a change in search strategy along the way. If you find a likely search term after you have searched several volumes, you know exactly where you have or have not checked the new term, even if your search is interrupted.

The record of sources checked can also help to avoid one of

	Al(OH)$_3$	Maalox	Mg(OH)$_2$	Benjamin, D. M.	McCormack, J. J.	Robinson, D. S.
IPA 10, #12 (6/30/73)						
Subject Index	878 1302[1] 1530	X[3]	881 1302[1]	—	—	—
Author Index	—	—	—	1302[4]	1302[4]	1302[4]
IPA 9, #24 (12/30/72)						
Subject Index	0[2]	0[2]	0[2]	—	—	—
Author Index	—	—	—	0[2]	0[2]	0[2]
IPA 9, #12 (6/30/72)						
Subject Index	0	0	1904	—	—	—
Author Index	—	—	—	0	0	0
IPA 8, #24 (12/30/71)						
Subject Index	0	X	0	—	—	—
Author Index	—	—	—	0	0	0

Figure 1. Interactions of Maalox or Its Components

Figure 1. Part of a sheet showing a *"Sources Checked"* record of a search through *International Pharmaceutical Abstracts* on interactions of Maalox or its components. (1) Note that abstract 1302 was the only one found under both aluminum and magnesium hydroxide. (2) An "0" indicates that nothing pertinent occurred under this heading. (3) An "X" shows that a cross reference to another heading occurred under this one. It is useful to continue to check headings which do not yield references because practices may differ in different years. (4) Authors checked were added because they had written the article cited in abstract 1302.

the most frequent errors in searching — failure to ascertain whether the files of sources checked are complete. Were all the issues of the periodical on the shelf when they were checked? If the abstract source was published in two or three volumes during the year, were indexes for all of them examined? Were there several different kinds of indexes to the abstracts, and

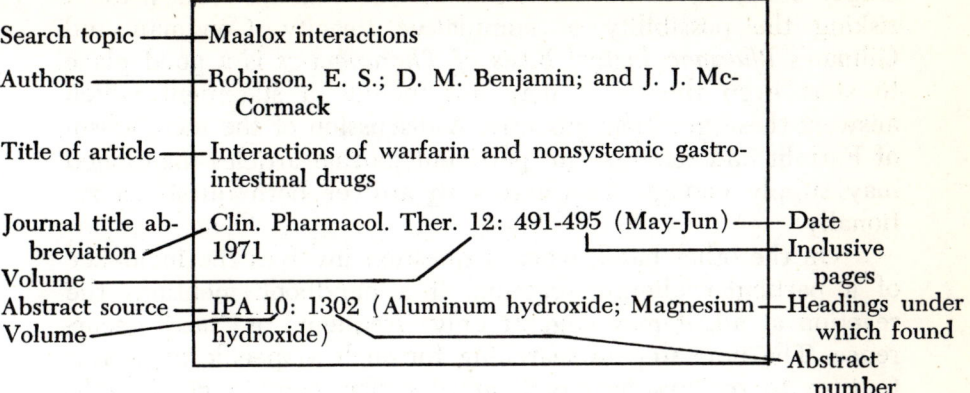

Figure 2. Card showing record of one *"Reference Found"* in the search through *International Pharmaceutical Abstracts*. (See Figure 1.)

were all the appropriate ones used? As a student I was highly insulted when I asked an experienced reference librarian a question and the first source she checked was the one I told her I had examined. I have since had many occasions to understand why she did so.

References found (see Figure 2) should include author, title, and full journal reference — journal name, volume number, inclusive pages and exact date of publication. This record should also show precisely where the reference was found, i.e., the name of the abstracting or indexing source, the volume, and the page or abstract number. A notation of the heading being checked at the time is a useful addition. Keeping each individual reference on a separate card allows the cards to be sorted in shelf order to find the original publication, and later to be rearranged into an appropriate order for bibliographies or footnotes (See Figure 2). For thesis bibliographies punch cards such as those discussed in Chapter 20 are convenient.

Selection and Use of Literature Sources (Search Strategy)

Besides the level of effort decided upon, other considerations will determine whether one will search in a handbook or text, a review, or an abstracting or indexing source. If a question concerns whether Farmlit should be administered on a full or empty stomach, or how often it can be administered without risking the possibility of cumulative toxicity, Goodman and Gilman's *Pharmacological Basis of Therapeutics* is a good place to start even though it may not include a statement which answers these questions directly. A discussion of the metabolism of Farmlit and reference to pertinent journal articles mentioned may supply enough information to answer both questions rationally.

On the other hand, when a question involves the incidence of a particular allergic reaction, if a handbook mentions the reaction at all, it may suggest only "frequent" or "rare" occurrence. The next step in searching for such a specific answer is to turn to reviews or recent articles that contain good bibliographies; however, they often do not give quantitative data even though they do mention the problem. If the question is important, you may have to do a thorough literature survey to find out how many papers have reported the reaction, and in those papers, the number of cases without reactions. If enough journal articles are checked, reasonable assumptions as to reaction incidence may be possible even though you never find in the literature a statement on the exact quantity.

This example demonstrates two instances in which one will use the abstracting and indexing services: when nothing adequate can be found in handbooks, texts, or reviews, and when quantitative data is needed. Another instance is that in which one wants negative data, for instance to assure oneself that no major adverse reactions to a drug have been reported. Obviously, abstracting and indexing sources will be used when exhaustive research is being done and when one needs very current information that would not yet be reported in handbooks and texts.

Decisions on which source to use will relate to the drug involved and the kind and depth of information wanted, as well as the scope, coverage, organization, and limitations of the services being considered. The latter matters will be described for individual publications in the next chapters.

Having decided which sources to use, you will next plan the places to look in the publication: which years will be checked and what terms looked under.

If you find that Farmlit was patented in 1959 and introduced to the market in 1962, you will know that papers on its synthesis and properties, on its animal pharmacology and toxicity, and on clinical investigations are likely to have appeared between the late 1950's and 1963, whereas most later articles may discuss new indications or clinical experience with adverse reactions. If you find key papers published from 1958 to 1963, you may be able to use *Science Citation Index* to find more recent articles that have cited the earlier ones, and hence will bring the earlier ones up to date.

Similarly, if you find recent pertinent articles, you may be able to do a "snowball search." This is simply the method of looking up all references cited in the first pertinent article and then in turn checking the papers referred to in these cited articles. It is a useful method and will be followed to some extent in nearly every search, but it cannot be used exclusively for an exhaustive search.

When looking for recent papers, check first the most recent annual cumulation of any source even though you know that a great deal has been published on the subject since the cumulated index was prepared. Checking for the larger volume will help you to find the correct headings, whereas you might labor through a number of monthly indexes thinking nothing was published on the subject in those issues before you realized you were just not looking in the place where pertinent material was listed.

You will know generally what terms are involved when you have familiarized yourself with your question, but what words you will actually check will depend on the kind of vocabulary in the particular service. Terms under which papers are listed in abstracting and indexing sources may come from a highly controlled, printed vocabulary; they may be standardized somewhat by following past practices in indexing; or they may be the author's terminology as it appears in the titles of articles. In any case, the problem is to find the right words to check and all the right ones.

To do so, one should remember three principles — multiplicity, specificity, and change.

1. *Multiplicity* means that one must think of all synonyms for each concept he wishes to find. In medicine you are likely to have to think of from two to four aspects for any concept — those related to a disease, its anatomic site, its etiology, and its therapy. For instance, if searching for antitubercular agents, one should check under all names for tuberculosis as well as

under antitubercular agents, *Mycobacterium tuberculosis*, and possibly even lungs.
2. *Specificity* is perhaps the biggest problem for an unsophisticated searcher. The scientist almost always assumes that anything he is looking for will be listed at the level of specificity at which he is thinking at the moment. For instance, if he wants everything on some aspect of heart diseases, it never occurs to him that he will have to look under myocarditis, congestive heart failure, arrhythmia, and literally hundreds of other names for heart diseases before he has found everything. In those abstracting and indexing systems in which individuals assign the terms, the indexer is invariably instructed to index to the most specific appropriate term only, putting under such broader terms as "heart diseases" only those articles which discuss many different diseases superficially. If the index service uses author's titles, you will have to look under all general and specific terms because you can't be sure how much the author generalized in his own thinking about his work when he decided on a title.
3. *Change* is one of the most constant characteristics of the human vocabulary. If you are searching in several volumes of an abstracting or indexing service, it is inevitable that new words will be invented for concepts that are at least somewhat familiar under earlier terms. "Drug interactions" are not completely different from "therapeutic incompatibilities." In *Medical Subject Headings*, the vocabulary for *Index Medicus*, new headings are listed at the front of each year's publication, and also in the *Cumulated List of New Medical Subject Headings 1963-1973*. These lists give the date of introduction of the term and the headings under which the same idea was listed previously. Every reference work must change from time to time in order to improve. Be alert to the possibility and if you suddenly find nothing under an index term you are using, do not assume without further checking that nothing on that subject was published that year.

Evaluation of the Search (Quality Control)

The pharmacist is familiar with the concept of quality control of the drug he dispenses but, although reliability of the information he provides is at least equally important, he may not think of controlling its quality. Assuming that he knows how to evaluate an individual article — touched on in Chapter 20 — he still may not know how to assure that he has found a good representation of current thinking on a problem. The technique for quality control of one's search method is simple. Take a selection of the best references you have found in one source (Source A), and check them by author to see if they are listed in a second abstracting or indexing publication (Source B). Now look under subject in Source B for the articles you know are there. If you don't find them all, keep trying other headings until you do. Did you have to use some new terms you didn't try in your search of Source A? If so, use these in Source A. In the process of your continuing search of both sources, watch for new references that you did not find in your first search. If they were in Source A, why didn't you find them?

If you don't find anything in either Source A or Source B under a heading you had not tried in your first search, you have the assurance that your technique was good and that you do have a good representation of current thinking on your problem, at least as it has appeared in publications.

CHAPTER **13**

SECONDARY SERVICES

One frequently hears the expression "secondary services," "secondary sources," or "secondary publications." A simple definition says that a "primary source" contains original reports and a "secondary source" points to and sometimes digests the information published elsewhere in a primary source.

Indexing services are secondary periodical publications which list each journal article or other publication by at least one aspect of the information it contains, using keywords, index terms, or subject headings. Usually the same original publication is listed under a number of different keywords. Abstracting services, in addition, provide a brief summary of the article — descriptive, informative, or merely indicative of the content. Sometimes authors' summaries are copied from the original journal. The abstract should give enough information about the article so that you will know whether or not to look at the original. For foreign-language articles, the abstract may have to serve in place of the article, although for important ones, a translation will probably be necessary.

Because all of the major secondary services are now published with the assistance of computers, each has spin-off products which will be described with the service. Some of these by-products are of greater interest to pharmacy than is the main publication. In addition, because the abstracts and indexes are in machine-readable format, their content for the last several years may be available through on-line services from various government and commercial organizations. Their data bases thus may be searched by computer, using a remote terminal to reach them through telephone lines. On-line searching in general will be discussed in Chapter 16, but some of the specific services will be mentioned with the publication involved.

This book is intended to stand alone, but because of the vast subject area involved — overlapping biology, chemistry, and medicine — many topics must be covered superficially. Some of the sources listed in Table 5 provide additional details about secondary services in the medical, biological and chemical fields.

The following description of secondary services does two things simultaneously: it gives for each publication information about its scope, coverage, terminology, and organization that will be useful in selecting the one to consult for a specific problem; and, where appropriate, it gives hints on the use of the various kinds of index represented in the different services. To avoid repetition in two separate sections, the name of a publication is identified in italicized heading at the beginning of its discussion. A special type of organization of an index being described is indicated in the margin. This approach should allow you to find information you want quickly, whichever aspect you need at a particular time.

International Pharmaceutical Abstracts

We have already mentioned *International Pharmaceutical Abstracts* as a means of keeping up with current literature, but its use as a tool for retrospective searching should not be overlooked. Besides covering pharmacy journals extensively, it includes good clinical articles, though fewer than are in *Index Medicus* or *Excerpta Medica*. Its organization and vocabulary are undoubtedly the easiest for the pharmacist to use. There are up to twenty-five sections in each issue which bring together abstracts on related topics.

An effort is made to use a controlled vocabulary, and cross-references are provided from a term that is not used to a term under which information on the subject will be found. However, if a new idea occurs, the editors can include it easily, since the rather small staff can pick up new terms with consistency. For instance, there is an entry for "laminar flow" in recent indexes although the concept does not appear in the 1975 *Index Medicus*. Official generic names for drugs are used in all cases.

Though there are only around 5,000 articles annually in *International Pharmaceutical Abstracts*, some of these will not be found in the more extensive abstracting publications. For instance, in a recent check of ten papers on pharmaceutical technology in *International Pharmaceutical Abstracts*, I was able to find five which had not appeared in *Chemical Abstracts* during four to five years after their publication. *International Pharmaceutical Abstracts'* coverage of pharmacy journals is generally better than that of much larger abstracting and indexing services.

In 1972 *International Pharmaceutical Abstracts* announced a more extensive complex of services from its computer data base, *IPA Information System*, including printed services, microform publications, customized searches and bibliographies, and computer tapes.

A useful by-product of this information system is *Drug Interactions-1* and *Drug Interactions-2*, compilations of all articles on drug interactions which appeared in *International Pharmaceutical Abstracts* during 1970 through 1972, together with their abstracts and an index to them.

A *Trade Name Cross Reference List* provides see references from the proprietary or trade name to the official nonproprietary or generic name, as well as a list of all trade names under the latter. The first issue covered January 1970 through December 1972.

International Pharmaceutical Abstracts is available on-line from 1970 onward as a part of the TOXLINE service.

Other Secondary Services in Pharmacy

Since *International Pharmaceutical Abstracts* began in 1964, one must consider its predecessors for retrospective searching in strictly pharmacy areas. Its immediate antecedent is "Comprehensive Bibliography on Hospital Pharmacy," which appeared in *American Journal of Hospital Pharmacy* and the preceding *Bulletin of the American Society of Hospital Pharmacists* in the January-February issues in 1951, 1953, 1955, 1957, and 1961 and the April 1965 issue. Prior to that, there was a very comprehensive publication, *Pharmaceutical Abstracts*, which was published by the American Pharmaceutical Association from 1935 through 1947.

The American Pharmaceutical Association's publication should not be confused with that issued by the University of Texas College of Pharmacy since 1957 and also called *Pharmaceutical Abstracts*. Originally named *Unpublished Abstracts of Articles on Pharmaceutical Subjects*, it contained abstracts submitted to *Chemical Abstracts* but rejected because of insufficient interest for that publication. It supplies many abstracts on the business and administrative aspects of pharmacy.

Chemical Abstracts

Chemical Abstracts is a weekly abstract periodical in which odd numbered issues consist of twenty sections on aspects of biochemistry and fourteen on organic chemistry. Even numbered issues include macromolecular chemistry, applied chemistry and chemical engineering, and physical and analytical chemistry. There are two complete volumes of twenty-six issues each year.

Chemical Abstracts is pre-eminent in its coverage. The proportion of its total field, chemistry, which it encompasses is higher than that for any other major secondary publication. Yet its scope in biology is limited to original work developing new biological aspects of a chemical. A large number of its abstracts of more than 300,000 papers and patents annually are drawn from relatively few sources. While an occasional article may come from any medical journal, one finds very few clinical papers in *Chemical Abstracts*. Hence, one must be cautious in making assumptions about the articles it will contain based on its journal coverage lists.

The organization of indexes to *Chemical Abstracts* is complex, offering many avenues of entry. Since the indexing is done from original papers, the indexes are sometimes more comprehensive than the abstracts. Frequently one may find a specific compound or other detail in the index which is not mentioned in the abstract.

KEYWORD
SUBJECT
INDEX

Each weekly issue has a Keyword Subject Index, an Author Index, a Numerical Patent Index, and a Patent Concordance. Since one will usually search in the total volumes rather than in individual issues, we will say of the weekly keyword indexes only that they are semistandardized, using title words, but normalizing them in certain instances. They usually do not list specific complex organic chemicals. They are used in the tape compilation known as *CA Condensates,* a data base from which on-line services are currently available.

CUMULATED INDEXES
Each volume has a cumulated subject index and several others. Besides the volume cumulations, indexes to the first 50 annual volumes were cumulated each ten years. After the Fifth Decennial Index, the collective indexes were cumulated every five years, and individual volumes are now issued semiannually. The cumulations add greatly to the efficiency of retrospective search in *Chemical Abstracts.*

Volumes 1-75 of *Chemical Abstracts* have single alphabetic subject indexes for both compounds and more general topics. With volume 76, the indexes were divided into a Chemical Substance Index and a General Subject Index. The latter "encompasses all of those headings which do not refer to specific chemical substances,"[1] including classes of substances, incompletely defined materials, applications, phenomena, reactions, biochemical and biological subjects (other than specific biochemicals), and common and specific names of animals and plants.

INDEX GUIDE — AUTHORITY LIST
For both these semiannual indexes, a very helpful Index Guide provides cross references to index entries. One should not use the Chemical Substance Index or the General Subject Index without first consulting the Index Guide for direction. For example, one does not find anything under "Drugs" in the General Subject Index, but an entry under "Drugs" in Index Guide leads one to "Pharmaceuticals," the heading used for nonspecific drug-related information in General Subject Index. Similarly, under "Effective charge" in Index Guide, there is a cross reference to "Electric charge, effective." Under some terms — for example, "Physiology" — there are "scope notes" to tell how that word is used in the subject indexes.

CHEMICAL SUBSTANCE INDEX — STANDARDIZED SUBJECT INDEX
Of greatest importance to the pharmacist is the fact that virtually no generic names for drugs appear in the Chemical Substance Index. He cannot say that a certain drug does not appear in *Chemical Abstracts* until he has looked at the Index Guide to find if it is there in a way he didn't anticipate. In Figure 3 is the page of the

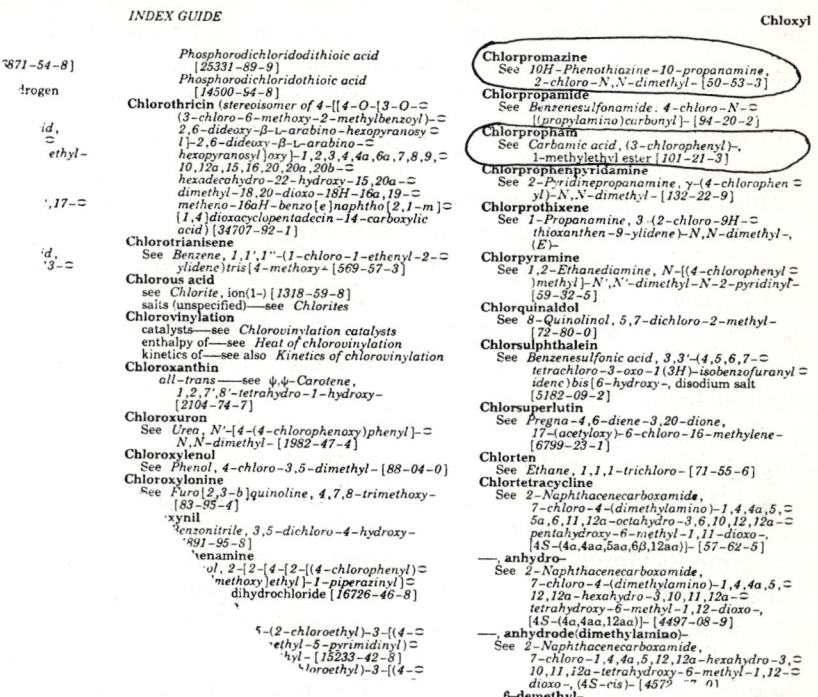

Figure 3. Part of a page from Index Guide which shows how chlorpromazine and other common names for substances are entered under their chemical names in the Chemical Substance Index of *Chemical Abstracts*. *Chemical Abstracts* 76: 167G (Jan.-June 1972).

Index Guide on which one finds the chemical name under which chlorpromazine is listed in the Chemical Substance Index.

The untrained user who is not familiar with chemical names may find it difficult in the Chemical Substance Index to zero in on a precise name among the complex of modifying phrases and positional indicators. It may help for him to understand a few points.

CHEMICAL NO-
MENCLATURE

First, a compound is named from its structure by very precise rules. The most recent published version appears in *Chemical Abstracts*, Volume 76, Index Guide (Chemical Abstracts Service,

The Ohio State University, Columbus, Ohio 43210, June 30, 1972. Pp. 21I-140I. Available separately as "Naming and Indexing of Chemical Substances for *Chemical Abstracts* during the Ninth Collective Period (1972-1976)" for $5.00.) The rules for the Ninth Collective Period were changed rather drastically from those used for the eighth and earlier collective indexes, and should be easier for the novice to understand.

The nomenclature remains systematic and some of the broad guidelines are the same. For instance, the primary part, or "parent name," under which a compound is found in the index, contains its most important "function" (acid, aldehyde, amine, etc.) sometimes combined with the largest or most complex ring or chain attached to it. Thus, in Figure 3, the ring, "phenothiazine," is combined with the chain, "propane," and the functional group, "amine," to make up the primary part of the chemical name for chlorpromazine. So that this parent name may form the "index entry," the name of the compound is inverted, with all other components appearing after a comma somewhat as one's given names appear after one's family name in the phone book. Insofar as they can be separated into independent entities, the substituents follow the parent name in alphabetic order, with numbers showing where they appear in the compound and brackets and parentheses indicating how modifiers are linked to their substituents. In the name for chlorpropham, for instance, in Figure 3, the parentheses around "3-chlorophenyl" tell us that the "chloro" radical is on the "phenyl" and not directly linked to "carbamic acid."

CHEMICAL INDEX ARRANGEMENT

The ordering of the compounds and subdivisions is described at the beginning of the Chemical Substance Index. Sometimes a long dash replaces the name of the parent compound, as is true in the entry which occurs just above the chemical name for chlorpromazine in Figure 4 (2-chloro-3,7-dimethoxy-N,N-dimethyl-10H-phenothiazine-10-propanimine (3930-46-9)). When there are many entries for one compound, as with chlorpromazine, they are divided by heading subdivisions — "analysis," "biological studies," "properties," "reactions," "compounds," "oxides," etc. Note that the words describing chemical compounds and derivatives follow the more general subdivisions in a second alphabet. (Note in column 3 of Figure 4 that "compounds" of chlorpromazine follow the "uses and miscellaneous"

2615CS JAN.–JUNE 1972–CHEM. SUBSTANCE INDEX 10*H*–Phenothiazine–10–propanamine., oxides

dimethylsulfamate [*35160-63-5*], P 25307n
iodide [*35160-58-8*], P 25307n
10*H*–Phenothiazine–10–ethanaminium
—, **2–chloro–*N*,*N*,*N*–triethyl–α–methyl–**
cyclohexylsulfamate [*35233-84-2*], P 25307n
iodide [*35233-83-1*], P 25307n
—, ***N*–(2–hydroxyethyl)–*N*,*N*,α–trimethyl–**
chloride [*35517-04-5*], metabolism of, biliary excretion in relation to, 41824j
—, ***N*,*N*,*N*,α–tetramethyl–**
methyl sulfate, cobalt thiocyanato complexes, 53861g
10*H*–Phenothiazine–10–ethanol [*7046-84-6*]
141316p
10*H*–Phenothiazine–2–methanol
—, **α–[[(1–methylethyl)amino]methyl]–** [*6887-21-4*]
sympatholytic activity of, 94939g
10*H*–Phenothiazine–10–propanamide [*35020-87-2*]
141316p
—, ***N*–[[(1–oxo–2–propenyl)amino]methyl]–**

electron–donating, 141316p
—, ***N*–[[(1–oxo–2–propenyl)amino]methyl]–** [*34613-05-3*], 141316p
10*H*–Phenothiazine–10–propanamine
—, **2–chloro–** [*2095-17-2*]
formation of, from chlorpromazine by liver microsomes, 21053d
—, **2–chloro–3,7–dimethoxy–*N*,*N*–dimethyl–**
monohydrochloride [*3930-46-9*], 113148s
10*H*–Phenothiazine–10–propanamine, 2–chloro–*N*,*N*–dimethyl– [*50-53-3*], **analysis**
detection of
of blood of cadaver, 136486q
in emergency toxicology, 149630g
transition metal thiocyanates for, 63175a
in urine, 649n
detn. of
photometric, 131574g
voltammetric, 144884h
identification of, 158417v
10*H*–Phenothiazine–10–propanamine, 2–chloro–*N*,*N*–dimethyl– [*50-53-3*], **biological studies**
acetylcholine release by cerebrum inhibition by, analgesia in relation to, 42031k
ACTH release and blood plasma corticosterone response to, scopolamine and trihexyphenidyl inhibition of, 108243q
adrenochrome interaction with, psychotropic action in relation to, 121504v
adsorption of, by brain, 94531t
aggressive behavior from brain stimulation response to, 21217k
aggressive behavior inhibition by, 68092f
aminobutyric acid metabolism by brain response to, 95239r
analgesic activity of, screening method in relation to, 107990u
anterior pituitary–hypothalamus system in response to, 108520c
antibody formation and reticuloendothelial phagocytosis response to, 171a
anticonvulsant activity of, in crowding stress–induced convulsions, 108134e
antihemolytic activity of, anesthesia in relation to, 135561y
apomorphine–induced behavior response to, dopamine metabolism in relation to, 41998u
arrhythmia from adrenaline in fluothane anesthesia inhibition by, 135819p
arrythmic action of, 56311b
artery contraction by ... hition by, 54572a

brain response to, 107968t
calcium metabolism in response to, 2161w
capillary permeability in anaphylaxis response to, 81279s
catechol amine metabolism response to, in brain, 121822x
central nervous system in response to, 121650q
convulsions from, convulsants in inhibition of, 21205e
corticosterone formation by adrenal cortex inhibition by, 121468m
cortisol of blood plasma in response to, endocrine system in relation to, 94825s
cyclic AMP of brain in response to, psychotropic activity in relation to, 94633c
diuretic activity of, dehydration–induced neurosecretory changes in relation to, 94619c
dopamine metabolism by brain in response to, cocaine in relation to, 94740k
dopamine metabolism by brain inresponse to, negro–striatal dopamine pathway in relation to, 135888k
dopaminergic receptors blockage by, in brain, antipsychotic activity in relation to, 21067m
enzymes of cortical synaptosomes in response to, 94721e
fatty acid metabolism by liver response to, 41976k
globulins of organs response to, 41961b
glucose metabolism by brain response to, 42024k
glutamine synthetase formation by brain in response to, 21254v
glycine absorption by nervous system inhibition by, 12535k
glycogen of brain hippocampus after administration of, 108159s
heart elec. and mechanical activity response to, potassium in, 10199e
histamine and serotonin of blood response to, 115k
histamine release by mast cell in response to, 68054v
hypertension from pain inhibition by, 54563y
hypothalamic neurosecretion in Shwartzman phenomenon in response to, 135886h
hypothermia from, creatine phosphokinase of blood plasma in, 94811j
hypothermia from clonidine antagonism by, 149016m
hypothermia from reserpine in response to, 68138a
hypothermia from reserpine reversal by, 68205v
hypothermia–recovery response to, 41888h
infections treatment by, dimebone and cyproheptadine in relation to, 94800e
iodide transport by thyroid gland inhibition by, after long–acting thyroid stimulator and TSH stimulation, 68416q
jaundice from, diagnosis of viral hepatitis and, 97572t
kidney cultures response to, as toxicity model, 54890c
kidney damage effect on activity of, 94727m
kidney function response to, antidiuresis in relation to, 42020f
in kidney preservation for transplantation, in ischemia, 108030t
lactate dehydrogenase isoenzymes response to, 69479y
lipids metabolism by adipose tissue in response to, histamine in relation to, 10307p
liver toxicity of naphthylisothiocyanate in response to, 81087c
lung blood vessel permeability and tonus in response to, 121717s
lysosome membrane stability of leukocytes and liver res... 30545t
mas...

Consult Index Guide
Before Using Index

rabbit fertility and growth response to, 10740z
reflex inhibition by, 41948c
respiraton in response to, 68063x
schizophrenia treatment with, Anatensol and Artane in relation to, 121928m
Shwartzman phenomenon in response to, hydroxycorticosteroids secretion by adrenal cortex in relation to, 135884f
skin allergy and brain elec. activity in response to, 54314t
sodium absorption inhibition by, erythrocyte ghosts as model for, 54268f
sound subthreshold levels in emotion in response to, 54448q
sympathetic response to brain stimulation inhibition by, 21223j
synaptic transmission response to, in brains, R 148627z
teratogenesis in relation to, 136501r
thrombus lysis response to fibrinolytic agents and, 121872p
tissue catecholamines in response to, reserpine in relation to, 135858a
toxicity of, in albinism, 121831z
trace elements metabolism in response to, 81072u
tranquilizing activity of, in horses, 54417d
vision distortion adaptation response to, 108268b
10*H*–Phenothiazine–10–propanamine, 2–chloro–*N*,*N*–dimethyl– [*50-53-3*], **properties**
crystal structure of, 98981n
dipole moment of, 126194d
mass spectrum of, 59548g
mass transfer of, between cyclohexane and water, effect of pH and resolvation rate on, 129408n
solv. of, tablets, 103680v
10*H*–Phenothiazine–10–propanamine, 2–chloro–*N*,*N*–dimethyl– [*50-53-3*], **reactions**
with peroxidase, free radical formation in, 135518q
reaction of
with Edecrin, 158277z
with mol. oxygen, 3159p
with surfactants, 103689e
10*H*–Phenothiazine–10–propanamine, 2–chloro–*N*,*N*–dimethyl– [*50-53-3*], **uses and miscellaneous**
corticosteroids detn. in urine interference by, 22654n
in detn. of iron, 80603f
10*H*–Phenothiazine–10–propanamine, 2–chloro–*N*,*N*–dimethyl–, compounds
compd. with 2,5–dimethyl–2,5–cyclohexadiene–1,4–dione (1:1) [*36459-21-9*], equil. const. and transition energy for, 112498u
monohydrochloride [*69-09-0*]
acetylcholine release by cerebral cortex inhibition by, 94569m
anesthesia from chloral hydrate and magnesium sulfate in response to, 10339a
behavioral disruption from levallophan in response to naloxone and, 94814n
behavior and sleep response to, chlordiazepoxide in relation to, 149035s
behavior response to, 121693f
behavior response to amphetamines and ephed... tment with, 1081...
beh... fter tre...

Figure 4. Part of a page from Chemical Substance Index which shows references to abstracts of papers on chlorpromazine (10*H*-Phenothiazine-10-propanamine, 2-chloro-N,N-dimethyl- (50-53-3)) in *Chemical Abstracts* 76: 2615CS (Jan.-June 1972).

subdivision.) After the bold-faced compound name and subdivision are found aspects of individual papers listed in "modifications," again alphabetically.

SPECIFIC COMPOUNDS RELATED TO A SINGLE DRUG

Remember that there are separate listings for an acid or base and its salts. In the "compounds" subdivision for chlorpromazine in Figure 4, the monohydrochloride is listed with a separate registry number (69-09-0), because some authors specified chlorpromazine hydrochloride. Since the pharmacist is usually interested in the drug whether or not a salt is indicated, he must look both places — under the primary chemical and under "compounds" toward the end of the listings. Similarly, a note in Index Guide under Glutamic acid (6899-05-4) indicates that "the *L*-isomer (56-86-0) has been assumed unless otherwise stated in the original document." However, the synthetic glutamic acid is indexed at *DL*-Glutamic acid (617-65-2), and there is also, of course, *D*-Glutamic acid (6893-26-1). One could theoretically find mono- or disodium salts at any of these entries.

In earlier indexes, if one author referred to *p*-hydroxy-acetanilide and another to hydroxyacetanilide, one paper appeared under "Acetanilide, hydroxy-," and the other under "Acetanilide, *p*-hydroxy-" even though the same compound was intended. Since this is a chemical, not a drug index, there could be intervening entries for "Acetanilide, *m*-hydroxy-" and "Acetanilide, *o*-hydroxy-" even though the pharmacist knows that acetaminophen, the *p*-hydroxy- analog, is the one that is often called merely hydroxyacetanilide in the medical literature. Hence it is important to check index entries near that of the exact compound to see if there are less specific names which are really synonyms.

With the introduction of more systemic indexing in Volume 76, some names have become inordinately long and complex. To assist the searcher, *Chemical Abstracts* has added some italicized generic names in parentheses immediately preceding their registry numbers. For instance, when one is looking for digitoxin, whose chemical name occupies five lines, one should locate the area where names begin as it does (Card-20(22)-enolide, 3-[(0-2,6-dideoxy- . . .) and then rapidly scan all such names to find the generic listing (*digitoxin*).

ABSTRACT NUMBERS

Finally, to understand the indexes, it is helpful to know how *Chemical Abstracts* refers in them to abstracts. In recent volumes, there is a different number for each individual abstract, but until 1966, columns — not abstracts or pages — are referred to by numbers which are followed by letters indicating, like map coordinates, the part of the column on which the reference to a compound or other indexed subject appears. In these column references, an abstract sometimes covers several lettered sections, but the letter in the index directs the user to the precise part of the abstract of interest to him. Capital letters precede

some of the numbers in the indexes. These can be interpreted as follows:
- B: the numbers direct one to a reference for a book
- P: the numbers direct one to a reference for a patent
- R: the numbers direct one to a reference for a review article.

Besides the two subject and the author indexes, *Chemical Abstracts* contains a Numerical Patent Index and several others which serve as cross references to those just mentioned — a Patent Concordance, a Formula Index, an Index of Ring Systems, and a Registry Number Index.

PATENT CONCORDANCE
Chemical Abstracts covers literally every chemical patent published throughout the world. In many instances, it relies on its concordance to lead from one patent to its equivalents in other countries, after the one first granted or listed has been abstracted fully.

FORMULA INDEX
The Formula Index is a way of finding a compound when one is unable to name the chemical oneself or find it through a synonym in the Index Guide. One simply calculates the molecular formula from the structure and looks for it in the Formula Index. The arrangement is primarily by increasing number of carbon atoms, and within compounds with the same number of carbons, by increasing number of hydrogens. When compounds contain other atoms, these follow carbon and hydrogen in alphabetical order, with subarrangements for each atom by increasing numbers of that atom. Under the specific molecular formula are found the names of all the different chemicals with that formula, its salts, complexes, etc., together with either abstract numbers or a reference to the Chemical Substance Index. In Figure 5, the molecular formula for chlorpromazine, $C_{17}H_{19}ClN_2S$, is followed by three entries for chlorpromazine, the primary chemical, its compound with another chemical, and the monohydrochloride, each with a separate registry number. The fourth entry is for an entirely different chemical, a thiourea, which happens to have the same molecular formula.

INDEX OF RING SYSTEMS
The Index of Ring Systems makes it possible to translate from the molecular formula of a ring to its name and the names of compounds which contain that ring. For example under C_5N, one finds not only "pyridine" and "piperidine" — the names for the

unsaturated and saturated rings — but also 16,28-Secosolanidane and Mocimycin — substances which contain the ring.

REGISTRY NUMBER INDEX

What is the Registry Number Index? A registry number is an "idiot" number (one assigned serially without any intrinsic meaning) which designates a computer record of a compound's structure. In the computer, every atom and every bond of the compound is "registered" to show its relationship to every other part of the compound, so that if ethers and esters related to acetaminophen are the subjects of a search, one can ask for all acetanilides with an oxygen in the *para* position, whether or not there is a substituent on the oxygen, or one can further specify that the substituent on the oxygen should be carbon. This compound can be searched for in the computer to obtain a list of registry numbers. The Registry Number Index simply provides the compound name in the instances in which one has found a registry number first. It was started with Volume 71 in 1969 and each volume thereafter covers registry numbers of compounds in the two annual *Chemical Abstracts* volumes each year. A cumulative *Registry Handbook-Name Section* covering two million compounds registered from 1965 through 1971 (Volumes 62-75) is planned for publication in the near future.

In addition to the *CA Condensates* on tape already mentioned, Chemical Abstracts Service distributes tapes of its semi-annual subject indexes in several formats, including the *CA Integrated Subject File,* which corresponds closely to its volume indexes, and the *CA Subject Index Alert,* which is issued biweekly. *Chemical-Biological Activities (CBAC),* contains the abstracts from the sections of *Chemical Abstracts* most pertinent to biology, as well as registry numbers, molecular formulas and names for the chemical substances discussed. These tape services are used by data centers and industrial firms and *CBAC* is a part of the TOXLINE on-line service.

For an overview of the printed indexes, one should refer to the first weekly abstract issue of each volume of *Chemical Abstracts.* For all services and publications, there is a pamphlet, *Information Services,* available from Chemical Abstracts Service, the Ohio State University, Columbus, Ohio 43210.

Current Abstracts of Chemistry and Index Chemicus

Another major index to chemistry is *Current*

SECONDARY SERVICES   123

JAN.-JUNE 1972-FORMULA INDEX $C_{17}H_{19}N$

-2,3-◯ $C_{17}H_{19}ClIrN$ Methanone, (3-chloro-4,7,7-trimethylbicyclo[2.2.◯
-4], 98583j   Iridium, chloro[(1,2,5,6-η)-1,5-cyclooctadiene]◯   1]hept-2-en-2-yl)phenyl-
lbutoxy)-   (quinoline)- [36671-12-2], 113359m   (-)- [35644-66-7], 85930v
                         $C_{17}H_{19}ClNO$ $C_{17}H_{19}ClO_2$
 methyl-   Oxazolidinium, 5-(4-chlorophenyl)-3,3-◯   Benzene, 1,1'-[(2-chloro-1-methylethylidene)◯
                              dimethyl-2-phenyl-   bis(oxymethylene)]bis- [35219-75-1], P
 ethoxy-◯   cis-,tetrafluoroborate(1-) [34880-02-9], 24570f   85419k
 448f $C_{17}H_{19}ClN_2$ $C_{17}H_{19}ClO_4$
 hexyl)-   1H-1,4-Benzodiazepine, 7-chloro-1-ethyl-2,3,4,◯   Naphtho[1,2-b]furan-2(4H)-one, 8-(acetyloxy)-◯
                              5-tetrahydro-5-phenyl- [35250-09-0], P   6-chloro-5,5a,6,7-tetrahydro-2,5a,9-◯
 ohexyl)-   46228c   trimethyl-
                           1,2-Ethanediamine, N'-[(4-chlorophenyl)◯   (5aR-cis)- [35087-66-2], 14735z
                              phenylmethylene]-N,N-dimethyl-   —, 8-(acetyloxy)-6-chloro-5,5a,6,7-tetrahydro-◯
 —   [35019-63-7], 34068n   3,5a,9-trimethyl-
 5887-92-4], $C_{17}H_{19}ClN_2O$ (5aR-trans)- [35087-64-0], 14735z
                           Benzenamine, 4-chloro-2-(4-morpholinylpheny◯ $C_{17}H_{19}Cl_2F_3N_2O_3$
 35887-91-3],   lmethyl)- [24855-26-3], P 99683d   1H-Benzimidazole, 5,6-dichloro-1-[[(octyloxy)◯
                         $C_{17}H_{19}ClN_2OS$ carbonyl]oxy]-2-(trifluoromethyl)-
 ◯   10H-Phenothiazine-10-propanamine,   [35649-77-5], P 59629j
 yphenyl)-   2-chloro-N,N-dimethyl- $C_{17}H_{19}Cl_2N_3O_5S$
                              N-oxide [1672-76-0], 21053d, 135494d   Pentanediamide, 2-amino-N,N'-bis[3-◯
 ◯   5-oxide [969-99-3], 21053d, 122322w, 148758t   (aminosulfonyl)-4-chlorophenyl]-
 492-13-8],   5-oxide, monohydrochloride [33870-13-2],   (S)- [35726-73-9], 113513g
                              94472z $C_{17}H_{19}Cl_2O_4P$
                              5-oxide, monohydrochloride [316-07-4], 94459a   Phosphoric acid
                           10H-Phenothiazin-3-ol, 8-chloro-10-[3-◯   bis(4-chlorophenyl)methyl diethyl ester
                              (dimethylamino)propyl]- [2095-62-7],   [34875-71-3], 59100e
                              135514k $C_{17}H_{19}Cl_2PPt$
 -4-◯ $C_{17}H_{19}ClN_2O_2$ Platinum, dichloro[[(4,5-η)-4-pentenyl]◯
                           Urea, N'-[3-chloro-4-[(4-methylphenyl)   diphenylphosphine-P]- [12094-85-8],
 l77e   methoxy]phenyl]-N,N-dimethyl-   141009r
 -6-◯   [34797-86-9], P 14150e $C_{17}H_{19}Cl_3N_2O_5S$
 14-3],   —, N-(4-chlorophenyl)-N'-[5-(1,1-◯   Carbonic acid
                              dimethylethyl)-2-hydroxyphenyl]-   1-methyl-1-[[4-oxo-3-[(phenylacetyl)amino]-◯
                              [25847-85-2], P 35218y   2-azetidinyl]thio]ethyl 2,2,2-trichloroethyl
                         $C_{17}H_{19}ClN_4O_2$ ester, (3R-cis)- [35935-90-1], P 99828e
 ◯   1-Piperazinecarboxylic acid, 4-[(6-chloro-1,3-◯   1-methyl-2-[[4-oxo-3-[(phenylacetyl)amino]-◯
 992-13-6],   dihydro-1-oxo-2H-inden-2-ylidene)methyl]-   2-azetidinyl]thio]ethyl 2,2,2-trichloroethyl
                              ethyl ester [34924-76-0], P 72549c   ester [35639-76-0], P 99989r
                         $C_{17}H_{19}ClN_2O_4S$ $C_{17}H_{19}Cl_3N_3OP$
 -dihydro-   Acetamide, N-[2-(chloroacetyl)-3,3-dimethyl-◯   Phosphorodiamidimidic chloride, N''-(2,2-◯
 26n   7-oxo-4-thia-1-azabicyclo[3.2.0]hept-6-yl]-◯   dichloro-1-oxopropyl)-N,N'-bis[2-◯
 osyloxy)◯   2-phenoxy-   methylphenyl)- [35232-03-2], 72149x
 ], 44006e   [2S-(2α,5α,6β)]- [34707-40-9], 14420t, P   —, N''-(2,2-dichloro-1-oxopropyl)-N,N'-bis◯
                              14556s   (3-methylphenyl)- [35232-04-3], 72149x
 yclopropyl)thio]-   Benzamide, N-[1-(4-chlorophenyl)ethyl]-4-◯   —, N''-(2,2-dichloro-1-oxopropyl)-N,N'-bis◯
                              methoxy-3-[(methylamino)sulfonyl]-   (4-methylphenyl)- [35232-05-4], 72149x
 enyl)thio]-   [35600-84-1], P 112932f   —, N''-(2,3-dichloro-1-oxopropyl)-N,N'-bis◯
                           4-Thia-1-azabicyclo[3.2.0]heptane-2-carboxylic   (2-methylphenyl)- [36076-30-9], 153295u
 cin,   acid, 3,3-dimethyl-7-oxo-6-◯   —, N''-(2,3-dichloro-1-oxopropyl)-N,N'-bis◯
 -5], 71576x   [(phenylacetyl)amino]- [2S-(2α,5α,6β)]-   (3-methylphenyl)- [36076-31-0], 153295u
                              chloromethyl ester [34573-47-2], P 3844h, P   —, N''-(2,3-dichloro-1-oxopropyl)-N,N'-bis◯
                              14535j   (4-methylphenyl)- [36076-32-1], 153295u
 150-02-3], $C_{17}H_{19}ClN_2O_5S$ $C_{17}H_{19}Cl_3N_3O_2P$
                           4-Thia-1-azabicyclo[3.2.0]heptane-2-carboxylic   Phosphorodiamidimidic chloride, N''-(2,2-◯
 0-13-3],   acid, 6-[[2-(5-chloro-2-thienyl)-3-methyl]-◯   dichloro-1-oxopropyl)-N,N'-bis(2-◯
                              1-oxo-2-butenyl]amino]-3,3-dimethyl-7-oxo-   methoxyphenyl)- [35232-06-5], 72149x
 14-4],   monopotassium salt, [2S-(2α,5α,6β)]-   —, N''-(2,2-dichloro-1-oxopropyl)-N,N'-bis◯
                              [35145-47-2], 10182u   (3-methoxyphenyl)- [35232-07-6], 72149x
 -95-5], $C_{17}H_{19}ClN_2O_5S$ —, N''-(2,2-dichloro-1-oxopropyl)-N,N'-bis◯
                           Benzoic acid, 3-(aminosulfonyl)-2-(butylamino)-◯   (4-methoxyphenyl)- [35232-08-7], 72149x
                              5-chloro-4-phenoxy- [35989-33-4],   —, N''-(2,3-dichloro-1-oxopropyl)-N,N'-bis◯
 omethyl]◯   108226m   (2-methoxyphenyl)- [36076-33-2], 153295u
 ], P 87290h   4-Thia-1-azabicyclo[3.2.0]heptane-2-carboxylic   —, N''-(2,3-dichloro-1-oxopropyl)-N,N'-(3-◯
                              acid, 3,3-dimethyl-7-oxo-6-◯   methoxyphenyl)- [36076-34-3], 153295u
 3-◯   [(phenoxyacetyl)amino]- $C_{17}H_{19}Cl_3O$
                              chloromethyl ester, [2S-(2α,5α,6β)]-   Methanone, phenyl(2,3,3-trichloro-4,7,7-◯
 03-0], 24570f   [34573-26-7], P 3844h   trimethylbicyclo[2.2.1]hept-2-yl)-
                         $C_{17}H_{19}ClN_2O_6S$ [35644-67-8], 85930v
 1-◯   4-Thia-1-azabicyclo[3.2.0]heptane-2-carboxylic $C_{17}H_{19}Cl_3O_5$
 nyl)-   acid, 6-[(4-chloro-2,6-dimethoxybenzoyl)◯   Carbonic acid
                              amino]-3,3-dimethyl-7-oxo-   2,4,5-trichlorophenyl 1,7,7-trimethylbicyclo[2.◯
                              monosodium salt, [2S-(2α,5α,6β)]-   2.1]hept-2-yl ester, exo-(±)- [34771-92-1], P
 2-carboxylic   [36546-54-0], 150446h   4160u
 enylpropyl)- $C_{17}H_{19}ClN_3S$ $C_{17}H_{19}FNO_2$
                           10H-Phenothiazine-10-propanamine,   Pyridinium, 1-[3-[2-(4-fluorophenyl)-1,3-◯
 150442d,   2-chloro-N,N-dimethyl- [50-53-3]. See   dioxolan-2-yl]propyl]-
                              Chemical Substance Index   chloride [35751-84-9], P 99534f
                              compd. with 2,5-dimethyl-2,5-◯ $C_{17}H_{19}FN_4O_2$
 rboxylic   cyclohexadiene-1,4-dione (1:1) [36459-21-9], Carbamic acid, [2-amino-6-[(5-fluoro-2,3-◯
 nzoyl)-   112498u   dihydro-1H-inden-1-yl)amino]-3-pyridinyl]-◯
                              monohydrochloride [69-09-0]. See Chemical   ethyl ester, monohydrochloride [30903-20-9], P
                              Substance Index   14357c
                           Thiourea, N-[2-(4-chlorophenyl)ethyl]-N'-(3-◯ $C_{17}H_{19}H_{17}N_2OS$
                              4-dimethylphenyl)- [35787-48-5], 107932b   Ethanaminium, N-(2-carboxyethyl)
                         $C_{17}H_{19}ClN_3S_2$

Figure 5. Part of a page from Formula Index which shows entries under the molecular formula for chlorpromazine, $C_{17}H_{19}ClN_2S$. *Chemical Abstracts* 76: 1095F (Jan.-June 1972).

STYLIZED
ABSTRACTS
Abstracts of Chemistry and Index Chemicus, produced by Institute for Scientific Information (ISI, which also publishes *Current Contents* and *Science Citation Index*). Initiated as *Index Chemicus,* a guide to newly synthesized compounds, it now covers all chemical papers in a core of about a hundred journals, and selections from others up to the 2,500 periodicals reviewed for ISI's *Science Citation Index*. It provides prompt, stylized abstracts, with reaction diagrams and structural formulas, in addition to authors' summaries. The emphasis on the new is continued by a listing in each weekly issue of labeled compounds, new syntheses and new reactions, and by underlining of new compounds in the stylized abstracts. Each issue also contains an Author Index, a List of Journals Covered, a Rotated Molecular Formula Index, and a Compound Name Subject Index. The latter is based on author terminology and is not necessarily the preferred systematic chemical name. However, a systematic approach to structure can be found in the separate *Chemical Substructure Index.*

ROTATED WIS-
WESSER LINE
NOTATION
INDEX
Chemical Structure Index; Substructure Index to Current Abstracts of Chemistry and Index Chemicus provides a means to search manually for certain aspects of the structure of a compound. It uses the Wiswesser Line Notation (WLN), a system for representing a structural formula in a continuous line by means of letters, numbers, and symbols which are defined in each issue. Further information on the notation can be obtained in *The Wiswesser Line-Formula Chemical Notation,* as revised by Elbert G. Smith in collaboration with a group of users (McGraw-Hill Book Co., 1221 Avenue of the Americas, New York, N.Y. 10020). The WLN is useful because it is concise, it designates each individual compound uniquely (except for stereoisomers), and the symbols are meaningful, so that all compounds containing certain structural features can be brought together. In the *Chemical Substructure Index,* the notations are rotated in a manner similar to that described in detail for the *Biological Abstracts* index. Thus efficient substructure searches are possible in the publication as well as on computer tapes.

Index Medicus and MEDLARS

Probably the broadest literature coverage of use to today's

pharmacist is found in the National Library of Medicine's *Index Medicus*. Around 225,000 articles from 2,300 journals are indexed annually for *Cumulated Index Medicus*, which interfiles the twelve monthly issues of *Index Medicus*. There are no abstracts, only author, title, and serial citations. The vocabulary used to index these periodical articles is more highly controlled than those of any of the other abstracting and indexing services here discussed.

STANDARDIZED VOCABULARY
Only those words listed as major descriptors (or main headings) in *Medical Subject Headings*, the guide to its vocabulary, are used as access terms in *Index Medicus*. *Medical Subject Headings* is issued annually as Part 2 of the January Index Medicus. Among medical librarians, it is commonly referred to by the acronym "*MeSH*." (Frustrated chemists and pharmacists occasionally say that stands for methyl mercaptan!) In spite of the problems of a rigidly controlled vocabulary, *MeSH* is an invaluable guide to the wealth of literature to be found in *Index Medicus*.

The major reason it is important to use *MeSH* is that the cross references and tree structures it contains do not appear at all in the monthly *Index Medicus* and only partially in its annual *Cumulated Index Medicus*. If you have an opportunity to search the on-line system, MEDLINE, the computer will recognize only the standardized terms found in *MeSH*. If you disregard the cross references and tree structures, you will miss many papers of importance.

MeSH is composed of two main sections: the Alphabetic List and the Categorized Lists (in "tree structure," or hierarchical format after 1974).

ALPHABETICAL LIST
In the Alphabetical List, you will find all of the headings that appear in *Index Medicus* and a number of others which serve as guides to *Index Medicus*' major descriptors (or main headings). In addition, the descriptor entries provide the numbers under which they are found in the Categorized Lists. There are three kinds of cross references showing the relationships of the major descriptors (1) to other major descriptors; (2) to synonyms; and (3) to minor descriptors. Minor descriptors do not appear in *Index Medicus* but refer to major ones where papers on their subject are found. In effect, the cross references define the mean-

ings of the major descriptors as they are used in *Index Medicus*. Let's look at examples of each kind.

SEE RELATED CROSS REFERENCES (AND XR's)

A *See related* cross reference alerts you to the fact that there may be material of interest to you under another major descriptor. For example, under HEAT, there are *See related* references to CALORIMETRY, DESERT CLIMATE, TROPICAL CLIMATE, and WATER POLLUTION, THERMAL. Although you would be unlikely to want papers on calorimetry and desert climate at the same time, when you look under HEAT, it is quite possible that references under one or two of the other terms in *Index Medicus* will also be important to your current interest. Under each of the headings referred to, there is an XR, or "backwards cross reference" — e.g., CALORIMETRY XR HEAT — showing when you are looking at CALORIMETRY that there is a *See related* reference to it at HEAT. These XR's sometimes help to remind you of other headings, even though you may not use them often. Certainly, it is not likely that you will want to look under HEAT when your primary interest is calorimetry.

SEE CROSS REFERENCES (AND X's)

The other two kinds of cross reference are from minor descriptors, under which no material is placed in *Index Medicus,* to major descriptors, under which any references to the subject will be found. The *See* reference is for synonymous relationships. PLANNED PARENTHOOD *See* CONTRACEPTION tells you that in *Index Medicus* you will find articles about planned parenthood under CONTRACEPTION. From that cross reference and the backward CONTRACEPTION X PLANNED PARENTHOOD reference, you know that for *Index Medicus'* purposes the two terms have the same or a closely related meaning.

SEE UNDER CROSS REFERENCES (AND XU's)

The *See under* cross reference guides you from a specific minor descriptor to a more general major one where material on the former will be found in *Index Medicus*. For instance HELIOTHERAPY *See under* SUNLIGHT tells us that articles on treatment of disease by exposing one's body to the sun will be found under SUNLIGHT, and SUNLIGHT XU HELIOTHERAPY informs us that in *Index Medicus* the term SUNLIGHT is defined to include its use in therapy.

CATEGORIZED
LISTS
Although all of these cross references are extremely useful in guiding you to the places where you will find material on your topic in *Index Medicus*, the Categorized Lists are even more essential to assure that you have found everything pertinent. If you are looking for all material on porphyrins, you will find its number, D11.557.727, in the Alphabetical List and turn to the D11 Category in the Tree Structures. There, following down to the 557's, and within them to the 727's, you will find:

PORPHYRINS	D11.557.727	
CHLOROPHYLL	D11.557.727.220	
HEMATOPORPHYRIN	D11.557.727.462	
HEME	D11.557.727.587	D8.176.425
HEMIN*	D11.557.727.587.462	

The asterisk tells you that HEMIN is a minor descriptor for a topic included in *Index Medicus* with the heading under which it is indented, HEME. You now know that to find all porphyrins you will have to look under four terms in *Index Medicus*: PORPHYRINS, CHLOROPHYLL, HEMATOPORPHYRIN, and HEME. Also, if you don't find as much as you need under HEMATOPORPHYRIN you can check PORPHYRINS for more general articles which may include material on hematoporphyrins incidentally.

You should be alert to the fact that other numbers in the tree lists, such as the D8.176.425 following HEME, refer to other parts of the tree. In D8, for example, HEME is included with COENZYMES. Though the added numbers in the Tree Structures may be truncated to save space, the Alphabetical List will always give the full number.

The major purpose of the numbers themselves for *Index Medicus* users is as finding guides to the Tree Structures. They are, however, very valuable in expediting MEDLINE searches. Indirectly, they also help to define terms just as the alphabetic cross references do. The fact that VEHICLES is in Category D26 (Chemicals and Drugs-Miscellaneous) immediately suggests that the subjects referrred to are not automobiles or bicycles. Similarly, PHARMACEUTIC AIDS is also in D26 rather than M (Named Groups (of Persons)). Even a nonpharmacist can thus deduce that pharmacy technicians are not intended.

In 1975 the Tree Structures were first intro-

ALPHABETIC CATEGORIZED LISTS

duced into the "public MeSH" associated with *Index Medicus*. Before that, there were alphabetic Categorized Lists which gave you essentially the same information, but there were fewer categories, and the numbers were different. Each term was arranged alphabetically at the margin and those terms immediately specific to it were indented under it. You had to look at each indented word to find if anything was, in turn, more specific to it. For example, in the former D10 Category, PORPHYRINS is indented under PIGMENTS among the PI's, but you have to turn to PORPHYRINS in the PO's to find that CHLOROPHYLL, HEMATOPORPHYRIN and HEME are specific to it and hence PIGMENTS as well.

CUMULATED LIST OF CHANGES

The practice of introducing a specific heading only after it is well established means that often one has to search under different terms in different years. Tolinase, for example, will be found under TOLAZAMIDE in 1973 and after, but under SULFONYLUREA COMPOUNDS in 1972 and under ANTIDIABETICS and/or SULFONAMIDES before that! Remember that the history of the headings is traced in *Cumulated List of New Medical Subject Headings 1963-1973* and that changes for a given year are described at the beginning of the *MeSH* in which they are introduced.

As with other indexes, there are a few "traps" to beware. DEXTRO AMPHETAMINE was separated and filed with the D's in 1963, and DEXTROTHYROXINE, in 1965, while LEVODOPA appeared under DOPA until 1975, when it was moved to the L's. Levothyroxine articles are still under THYROXINE in 1975. Salts are usually found with their parent compounds. Both phenobarbital and phenobarbital sodium are under PHENOBARBITAL.

QUALIFIERS (SUBHEADINGS)

It is easy to be overwhelmed and discouraged by the number of papers listed under an appropriate descriptor in *Cumulated Index Medicus*, particularly when you realize that it covers only one of several headings under which useful material may be found and only one of many years during which items of importance were published. Two elements under the major descriptor may help to speed the search. One is the qualifier or subheading. *Index Medicus* uses relatively few qualifiers and those have meanings that may seem arbitrary. Look at the Introduction to *MeSH* to find how they are defined. Remember that articles aren't written with descriptors and qualifiers in mind, and consequently several subheadings under one drug name may be equally appropriate for a single paper. For example, a paper on chlorpropamide may discuss both "therapy" and "administration & dosage." Usually both qualifiers appear in the computer files, but only one is used in the printed index. Sometimes a paper for which a number of subheadings would be appropriate is simply put "up front" without any qualifiers. Do not rely on the qualifiers slavishly. Instead of choosing a single one to look under, it may be wiser to choose those you can skip. For instance, if you are looking for something on dosage of chlorpropamide in adults, you may wish to check up front and under "therapeutic use," "poisoning," "metabolism," "adverse effects," and even "pharmacodynamics," as well as under "administration and dosage," but you will not be likely to find much on this subject among papers which are primarily on "chemical synthesis," or "isolation & purification."

ARTICLE ARRANGEMENT IN SUBJECT INDEX
Another way of speeding the search is to look for papers in English only. You can then skip titles with brackets which appear after the English-language articles under each subheading. Note also that the papers are ordered alphabetically by language after English. Within language, the arrangement is by journal title abbreviation.

Most of the drugs or chemicals you need to locate will be in *MeSH*, but let's try one that isn't listed there to see how you would find material on it in *Index Medicus,* and to review general search techniques. Let's assume you want to find anything that has been included in *Index Medicus* on clioxanide (Parke Davis' Tremerad®, also called CI 633, SYD-230, and CN-59,567). You already know it is 4'-chloro-3,5-diiodosalicylanilide and that it has been used as an anthelmintic to treat ovine or bovine fascioliasis.

First you should check the drug name and its synonyms. In this case, you do not find any name for clioxanide in the 1975 *MeSH*. Next try looking under its action group. If you are not sure what terms are available, you can start with the broad one, ANTHELMINTICS. Under it, in the 1975 *MeSH*, you will find a See related HEXYLRESORCINOL, which is of no interest for this purpose and an X VERMIFUGES — showing that ANTHELMINTICS and VERMIFUGES are considered to be synonymous.

There are also references from ANTINEMATODAL AGENTS and FILARICIDES — telling us that agents with these activities will appear in *Index Medicus* under ANTHELMINTICS — and, finally, an XR HELMINTHIASIS because there is a *See related* reference from that term to ANTHELMINTICS. You will not see terms for antitrematodal or antiplatyhelmintic agents, which are the groups under which antagonists to fasciola would fall, until you have checked the tree number for ANTHELMINTICS, D21.201. In the Categorized List under that number you will find ANTIPLATYHELMINTIC AGENTS, the term you will use for *Index Medicus* searching. But first you must check the specific compounds under ANTIPLATYHELMINTIC AGENTS as well as the group term, SCHISTOSOMICIDES. You note that none of the compounds are clioxanide or its synonyms. However, you should either determine that clioxanide is not active against *Schistosoma* or check the group term SCHISTOSOMICIDES as well as ANTIPLATYHELMINTIC AGENTS in *Index Medicus*.

Your search of ANTIPLATYHELMINTIC AGENTS will be frustrating because the term does not appear in *Index Medicus* before 1975. This fact should alert you to look in the front of the 1975 *MeSH* to see whether ANTIPLATYHELMINTIC AGENTS is a new heading; it is. You will find that items now listed under that heading were formerly placed under ANTHELMINTICS.

Your search of earlier *Cumulated Index Medicus* volumes for ANTHELMINTICS will yield an article on clioxanide in 1972. Depending on your interest in the diseases and organism, you will decide on whether you want to pursue the references under HELMINTHIASIS, FASCIOLIASIS, FASCIOLA HEPATICA, etc., but you will be unlikely to find additional articles on the drug itself.

You should be aware that you can also approach your compound from the chemical point of view, though usually less effectively than from that of its action. Beginning with January 1975, a new subheading — "analogs & derivatives" — became available for use with *Index Medicus*. This means that if the compound you are looking for can be considered to be a chemical analog or derivative of one already in *MeSH* you may find information on it under the latter. In the case of clioxanide, it has the same basic salicylanilide structure as does Yomesan® (the trade name for niclosamide — and incidentally, one of the few trade names you will find in *MeSH*, which customarily uses the generic name). Hence, you should check under YOMESAN/ analogs and derivatives, even though the substituents on the rings of the two compounds are rather different. If you are not familiar with the composition of the other anthelmintics in the tree structure, check them out to insure that none of them could be construed to be related to clioxanide, although in this case I can assure you that they would not.

The other method of checking for the chemical, and the only one to consider before 1975, is to find the closest major chemical group name in the D2 or D3 categories (Chemicals-Organic and Chemicals-Organic, Heterocyclic) and look for clioxanide under it. The closest "parents" happen to be SALICYLAMIDES or ANILIDES. You will find the same paper under ANILIDES as you found under ANTHELMINTICS. Some related compounds are under SALICYLAMIDES. I suggest that you check the action term first because it is easier, more direct, and more consistent.

Like other services, *Index Medicus* is produced by computer and it is only a small part of what can be drawn from MEDLARS (Medical Literature Analysis and Retrieval System). In MEDLARS, there are added to an article many index terms under which it does not appear in *Index Medicus*. Although most of the added terms can be found in the published *MeSH*, either as synonyms or as minor or major descriptors, there are a very few "check tags," and a number of geographic terms that can be searched only in the computer. Check tags describe aspects of a subject that are too general to be used as entries in *Index Medicus* — words designating "human," "male," "female," age groups, experimental animals, etc. With the exception of a few papers included for the *Index to Dental Literature* and the *International Nursing Index*, all articles in MEDLARS will appear under at least one major descriptor in *Index Medicus*.

RECURRING BIBLIOGRAPHIES
MEDLARS is used for several purposes. It is the source of about twenty recurring bibliographies — *Index to Dental Literature, International Nursing Index, Cerebrovascular Bibliography*, and *Toxicity Bibliography* among others, all of which are listed inside the back cover of each monthly issue of *Index Medicus*. It is also the source of several hundred printed "Literature Searches" on subjects expected to interest a wide audience. Some examples are:

L.S. No. 73-26. The hospital emergency room. January 1970 through June 1973. 194 citations.

L.S. No. 73-32. Hypertension: diagnosis, occurrence, and prevention (with emphasis on studies in the U.S.). January 1970 through July 1973. 216 citations in English.

L.S. No. 73-33. Doping and sports. January 1970 through August 1973. 46 citations.

Literature Searches are listed in the front of the monthly issues of *Index Medicus* and in a number of other publications. They may be obtained without charge from Literature Search Program, Reference Section, National Library of Medicine, 8600 Rockville Pike, Bethesda, Maryland 20014.

ON-LINE SECONDARY SERVICES

MEDLINE (MEDLARS On-Line) may be the most familiar and important by-product of MEDLARS. It is the data base which can be reached on-line at remote terminals in American medical schools as well as in many other hospital and medical libraries. Though there is a small charge, it is absorbed by some of the libraries. The MEDLINE data base consists of the citations from about 2,300 journals which have appeared in *Index Medicus* in approximately the past three years. There are supplementary files containing MEDLARS citations for preceding years and an SDILINE — all the citations for the current month of *Index Medicus* — for convenience in monthly alerting searches. Though the MEDLARS data base is more than ten years old, searches are usually limited to more recent files except by special arrangement.

Since the programs used to operate MEDLINE are very simple, you can easily learn the commands and conventions in an hour or two. Though it is more difficult to attain truly effective use of the vocabulary, that too is easier when you can see exactly how each article is indexed. While MEDLINE uses the same data as *Index Medicus* and the same *MeSH* vocabulary, it has the advantage that you can search on minor descriptors and their synonyms as well as the major descriptors required for *Index Medicus*. In addition, the Tree Structure numbers are primarily for use in computer searches. If I want all the material on hexosamines, I simply can ask the computer to EXPLODE D9.203.67.342 and in effect have it check all descriptors which contain that number (HEXOSAMINES or GLUCOSAMINE or

GALACTOSAMINE) with this simple request. In addition, you will remember that most articles are indexed under a few terms for *Index Medicus* and under many more for MEDLINE, though all are taken from the *MeSH* vocabulary. Thus, if I want all articles on hexosamines, even if they were discussed only briefly or in passing in the article, I will find them in MEDLINE, not in *Index Medicus*. I would encourage every pharmacy or other health science student to investigate MEDLINE if it is available in his school.

Excerpta Medica

Excerpta Medica has the advantage of providing the pharmacist with English-language abstracts of medical papers. Though its list of periodicals indexed is longer than that of *Index Medicus*, the number of articles covered is slightly lower because *Excerpta Medica* is more selective in including papers from the journals.

PUBLICATION IN PARTS
Excerpta Medica is directed primarily to individual physicians, and hence is broken down into sections which are in effect separate abstract publications. As a result, it is more difficult to use as a whole than is *Index Medicus*. One must first decide which publication is pertinent. Frequently more than one must be checked. There are nearly forty different titles, ranging from *Anatomy, Anthropology, Embryology and Histology* through *Anesthesiology; Cardiovascular Diseases and Cardiovascular Surgery; Pediatrics; Pharmacology and Toxicology;* and *Public Health, Social Medicine and Hygiene;* to *Urology and Nephrology*. Rather than browse among the shelves, one can use *A Guide to the Use of the Excerpta Medica Abstract Journals* (Excerpta Medica Foundation, 228 Alexander Street, Princeton, N.J. 08540, 1969). Under 4,000 topics for which one may be searching, the *Guide* lists the appropriate abstract journal to check.

Whereas *MeSH* contains fewer than 10,000 subject headings, under which references appear, *Excerpta Medica* has many more — estimates having ranged from 40,000 to 150,000. This means that in the *Internal Medicine* index, one may find material during different years under "Kidney diseases, acute," and "Acute kidney diseases." For a complete search, one has the advantage of section groupings within a volume. Turning to the body of the *Internal Medicine* abstracts, Section 15 on kidney diseases, one finds additional articles on acute kidney diseases which were apparently indexed under headings other than those mentioned. This ability to turn to the general subject area and browse is, indeed, a great aid to the researcher who is not quite sure what he is looking for.

Like other computer-based services, *Excerpta Medica* publishes a number of by-products, two of which are of particular interest to pharmacists: *Adverse Reaction Titles* — an index of all papers on untoward effects of drugs or chemicals — and *Drug Literature Index* — an index by generic name, trade name, and activity class to papers which involve drugs. Instead of abstracts, these publications provide titles followed by keywords.

Checking *Drug Literature Index* is probably the quickest way to find a collection of published papers on a drug that is not yet well enough known to be in *Index Medicus* or MEDLINE, as well as many European papers not found in those sources. The indexes are merely lists of headings followed by citation numbers without any indication of what aspect of the drug is discussed in a given paper. Consequently, they can be laborious to use when searching for well-known drugs. If one is looking for the relationship between two common drugs, however, the search can be accelerated by comparing the citation numbers under the two to determine what they have in common.

For several years, *Excerpta Medica* has distributed tapes called DRUGDOC to industrial organizations. In early 1975, Informatics Inc. made the current volume plus two previous years of *Excerpta Medica* available on-line.

Biological Abstracts and Bioresearch Index

Biological Abstracts and *Bioresearch Index* are published by BIOSIS (*Bio*Sciences Information Service of *Biological Abstracts*). They cover the whole field of biology very broadly and included more than 240,000 citations to original journal articles and similar materials in 1974. *Biological Abstracts* has supplied scientists with abstracts of original papers since 1926.

ABSTRACTS OF MEETING PAPERS AND OTHER UNUSUAL SOURCES

Instead of providing abstracts, *Bioresearch Index* is only an index, including citations for each paper plus the same kind of author and subject indexes as does *Biological Abstracts*. Like *Biological Abstracts*, *Bioresearch Index* covers the field of biology, but the form of material it includes differs from that in most of the other abstracting and indexing sources. It is definitely the best place to find listings of papers which were presented at meetings but may or may not have been published in journals. For instance, *Federation Proceedings* contains abstracts of around 3,000 papers presented each spring at the meeting of the Federation of American Societies for Experimental Biology. Only a part of these papers are ever published in journals, and sometimes the time lag between presentation at the Society meeting and publication in a primary journal is as much as three years. The only major source in which Federation papers are indexed other than in its own *Proceedings* issue is *Bioresearch Index*. Besides proceedings and abstracts of many other meetings, *Bioresearch Index* also indexes letters to the editor, state and local documents, such as experiment station reports, and other material that rarely finds its way into the mainstream of journal article publication.

ROTATED TITLE (KWIC) INDEX

To turn from their coverage to their organization, *Biological Abstracts* and *Bioresearch Index* are primarily indexed by the titles of cited articles, using the Keyword in Context (KWIC) method. This is also called the permuted title index method, even though, strictly speaking, the titles are rotated, not permuted. To use this index, one needs to know that the keyword or index term (listed alphabetically as in any other subject index) will be found in the middle of a column, with a part of the title in front of it and a part behind, depending on the amount of space available in the column. For example, a paper on "*Therapy* of *chronic bronchitis* with *isoproterenol*" would appear in the index under each of the italicized words, but different parts of the rest of the title would be shown with them, as follows:

py of chronic   bronchitis with isoproter
ol/Therapy of   chronic bronchitis with i
onchitis with   isoproterenol/Therapy of
soproterenol/   Therapy of chronic bronch

Note that in each case at least one word of the total title is missing, that each keyword appears after the blank space in the center of the column, and that, if the title is completed before the end of the column, it is begun again after a slant line with its first word.

Though the principle is simple, the execution is

TERMS ADDED TO TITLES   a little more complex because *Biological Abstracts* editors add keywords to the end of the title. These words may relate to organisms, drugs, chemicals, instrumentation, methodology, geographic location, etc. With respect to drugs, the names of those significant to the cited paper will appear whether or not they were in the title. For example, the underlined items in both Figures 6 and 7 refer to a paper by K. Kuschinsky, "Morphine Catalepsy in the Rat: Relation to Striatal Dopamine Metabolism" (*Eur. J. Pharmacol.* 19(1):119-122, 1972, abstract no. 62381). Because other drugs are discussed in the article, the editors added the terms: "Chlorpromazine," "Naloxone," "L Dopa," and "Apo morphine." In Figure 6 under "Dopamine," one observes the end of the title — beginning with the last two letters in "Rat" — followed by "Chlorpromazine and "N" — the first letter in "Naloxone." In Figure 7, although we find only the last two-and-a-third words from the title, we see more of the added words, including the complete names for two other drugs and the beginning of "Apo Morphine." Thus the title is rotated to be included more or less fully at a given point depending upon the position of the index word in the title and how many terms are added. Note in the top right hand of the first column in Figure 6 that there are several slash lines preceding the beginnings of titles, such as "Biochemic . . .," "Effect of . . .," and "Mode of . . . ."

Besides adding specific drug names, the editorial staff uses twenty-eight terms from *U.S. Pharmacopeia XVII* (1965) class names to identify the action of drugs mentioned. Thus either Lasix® or furosemide (whichever term is used in the paper) will be followed by "Renal-acting-drug" in the expanded title. (The hyphens cause "Renal-acting-" to be filed as one word following "Renal venous blood" in the alphabet.) Articles on furosemide will be found under "Renal-acting-drug" in the index regardless of which name for the drug was used by the author. Of course all other drugs classified by *U.S.P.* as renal-acting are interspersed in the same area of the index, so that one may get more than one wishes. When addition of keywords to a title causes a problem, because the whole title line becomes simply a list of drug names and activities with no indication of the subject matter of the paper, the simplest solution is to turn to the abstract.

Remember that use of this index depends upon

ACI–1900 DOPAMINE DORMANCY

TIM-DRUGS/ EFFECTS OF A	DOPAMINE BETA HYDROXYLASE INHIBITOR	33358
ROXYLASE INHIBITORS AND	DOPAMINE BETA HYDROXYLASE INHIBITORS	27723
OL RING DEHYDROXYLATION	DOPAMINE BETA HYDROXYLASE INHIBITORS	50786
NE TYROSINE HYDROXYLASE	DOPAMINE BETA HYDROXYLASE MONO AMINE	4439
EAN UPOGEBIA-LITTORALIS	DOPAMINE BETA HYDROXYLASE N METHYL T	14289
PURIFICATION PROCEDURE/	DOPAMINE BETA HYDROXYLASE OF BOVINE	48305
AIN AFTER INHIBITION OF	DOPAMINE BETA HYDROXYLASE PROBENECID	27727
IMIPRAMINE METAB-DRUGS	DOPAMINE BETA HYDROXYLASE RADIOACTIV	10103
DEHYDROGENASE FUMARASE	DOPAMINE BETA HYDROXYLASE TYROSINE H	32876
AMINES ATP CHROMOGRANIN	DOPAMINE BETA HYDROXYLASE/ BIOCHEMIC	54042
RENALINE NOREPINEPHRINE	DOPAMINE BETA HYDROXYLASE/ EFFECT OF	56967
MINE MONO AMINE OXIDASE	DOPAMINE BETA HYDROXYLASE/ MODE OF A	50882
GS 4 METHYL METARAMINOL	DOPAMINE BETA HYDROXYLASE/ ON THE DI	50793
AN RAT CARDIO VASC-DRUG	DOPAMINE BETA HYDROXYLASE/ THE CLINI	9891
ENALS STRENGTHENING THE	DOPAMINE BETA OXIDASE EFFECT DEPLETI	42772
METHYL ESTER METAB-DRUG	DOPAMINE BETA OXIDASE/ INVOLVEMENT O	59897
IC LIVER DISEASE WITH A	DOPAMINE BLOCKING AGENT PATHO PHYSIO	62175
CUMULATION OF TRITIATED	DOPAMINE BY ISOLATED BRAIN MITOCHOND	39024
E AND LOSS OF CARBON-14	DOPAMINE BY PLATELETS FROM CHILDREN	63390
NOL RESERPINE 6 HYDROXY	DOPAMINE CARDIO VASC-DRUGS/ THE FIXA	27522
IM-DRUGS NOREPINEPHRINE	DOPAMINE CENT-DEPRESS-DRUGS/ BEHAVIO	10141
NISTRATION OF 6 HYDROXY	DOPAMINE CENT-STIM-DRUG DIAZEPAM HAL	57002
THYL TYROSINE 6 HYDROXY	DOPAMINE CENT-STIM-DRUGS MONO AMINE	33297
XY TRYPTAMINE SEROTONIN	DOPAMINE CENT-STIM-DRUGS URETHANE CE	50885
TRICAL SELF STIMULATION	DOPAMINE CONTAINING NEURONS LOWER BR	4082
NETHYLAMINES PRECURSORS	DOPAMINE DOPA EPININE TYROSINE AMINO	22209
THE CAT NOREPINEPHRINE	DOPAMINE DOPA/ MONO AMINES IN THE CA	6814
VANILLIC-ACID EXCRETION	DOPAMINE EXCRETION DIAGNOSTIC TESTIN	67240
NEPHRINE NOREPINEPHRINE	DOPAMINE EXCRETION FLUOROMETRY/ CASE	32720
TEMATICS ACETYL CHOLINE	DOPAMINE FLOREYS FACTOR 1 GAMMA AMIN	50828
DRENALINE AND TRITIATED	DOPAMINE FROM FIELD STIMULATED CEREB	38974
ATOGRAPHY/ FORMATION OF	DOPAMINE FROM 3 METHOXY TYROSINE FAC	38892
YDROXYLATES TYRAMINE TO	DOPAMINE FRUIT PULP PHENOLS ASCORBIC	4802
TIM-DRUGS ISOPROTERENOL	DOPAMINE HALOPERIDOL PROPRANOLOL SCO	21714
TRITIUM NOREPINEPHRINE	DOPAMINE HEART LEVELS/ EFFECTS OF CH	29014
SE RAT RABBIT SEROTONIN	DOPAMINE HISTAMINE ELECTRON MICROSCO	30883
OMO VANILLIC-ACID DOPAC	DOPAMINE HOMOGENTISIC-ACID ALKAPTONU	29013
EM/ THE CONFORMATION OF	DOPAMINE HYDRO CHLORIDE NERVOUS SYST	9690
PMENTAL CHARACTERISTICS	DOPAMINE HYDROXYLASE EC-1.14.2.1 NOR	42203
ALTERATIONS INDUCED BY	DOPAMINE IN A GROUP OF CORONAROPATHI	62130
THE METABOLISM OF BRAIN	DOPAMINE IN HUMAN PARKINSONISM MOTOR	32786
EPHRINE EPINEPHRINE AND	DOPAMINE IN HUMAN URINE/ A FLUOROMET	7443
PATHECTOMY BY 6 HYDROXY	DOPAMINE IN THE ADULT RAT EFFECTS ON	50925
HEMODYNAMIC EFFECTS OF	DOPAMINE IN THE AWAKE DOG PROPRANOLO	44929
INJECTION OF 6 HYDROXY	DOPAMINE IN THE CAT SUBSTANTIA NIGRA	15459
METABOLISM OF CARBON-14	DOPAMINE IN THE DECAPOD CRUSTACEAN U	14289
DRUGS ON THE 6 HYDROXY	DOPAMINE INDUCED DEGENERATION OF ADR	68184
ING CAUSED BY 6 HYDROXY	DOPAMINE INDUCED RELEASE OF NORADREN	62473
SPECIFIC ANTAGONISM BY	DOPAMINE INHIBITORS OF ITEMS OF AMPH	57013
TIONS OF NOREPINEPHRINE	DOPAMINE ISOPROTERENOL AND 5 HYDROXY	21696
ENTS RAT NOREPINEPHRINE	DOPAMINE L ALPHA HYDRAZINO-ALPHA-MET	10153
WITH DOPA AND 6 HYDROXY	DOPAMINE L ALPHA HYDRAZINO-ALPHA-MET	57003
AMPHETAMINE METAB-DRUGS	DOPAMINE MACROAUTO RADIOGRAPHY/ NEUR	52758
N THE EGG METHY LAURATE	DOPAMINE MELANIZATION/ STUDIES ON VI	43697
RAT IN-VITRO 6 HYDROXY	DOPAMINE METAB-DRUG DL OCTOPAMINE DL	21691
N BRAIN AFTER 6 HYDROXY	DOPAMINE METAB-DRUG NORADRENALINE NO	56996
S PERIPLANETA-AMERICANA	DOPAMINE METAB-DRUG/ HORMONAL CONTRO	31750
AIN FOLLOWING 6 HYDROXY	DOPAMINE METAB-DRUGS ADENYL CYCLASE/	39013
OLAMINE RAT EPINEPHRINE	DOPAMINE METAB-DRUGS CEREBRO SPINAL	38594
THE QUAIL HYPOTHALAMUS	DOPAMINE METAB-DRUGS LUTEINIZING HOR	42839
AIN RESERPINE 6 HYDROXY	DOPAMINE METAB-DRUGS P TYRAMINE M TY	21692
MIDE ACTINOMYCIN D DOPA	DOPAMINE METAB-DRUGS PROTEIN SYNTHES	62383
RENALINE NOREPINEPHRINE	DOPAMINE METAB-DRUGS RADIOACTIVITY M	38892
IAA NOREPINEPHRINE AND	DOPAMINE METAB-DRUGS 5 HYDROXY TRYPT	27709
EFFECT OF TROPOLONE ON	DOPAMINE METABOLISM AND THE CATECHOL	45057
AT RELATION TO STRIATAL	DOPAMINE METABOLISM CHLORPROMAZINE N	62381
GY OF PARKINSONISM DOPA	DOPAMINE METABOLISM ENZYMES NOREPINE	61857
ETAMINE CENT-STIM-DRUGS	DOPAMINE METABOLISM NOREPINEPHRINE M	50940
OF 3 4 DI-O METHYLATED	DOPAMINE METABOLITES BY MAMMALIAN TI	27598
4-HYDROXY MANDELIC-ACID	DOPAMINE METANEPHRINE NORMETANEPHRIN	35729
AB-DRUGS NOREPINEPHRINE	DOPAMINE MONO AMINE OXIDASE DOPAMINE	50882
YPTAMINE NOREPINEPHRINE	DOPAMINE MONO AMINE OXIDASE/ INTERAC	21699
RESCENCE METHOD HYDROXY	DOPAMINE NERVE GROWTH FACTOR/ HISTOC	230
ENTATION NOREPINEPHRINE	DOPAMINE NEURO ENDOCRINE/ CHANGES	
THE TUBERO INFUNDIBULAR	DOPAMINE NEURONS BLOCKADE OF C	
THE TUBERO INFUNDIBULAR	DOPAMINE NEURONS RAT 2 BROM	
AND CATECHOLAMINES RAT	DOPAMINE NORADRENALINE NO	
N RAT BRAIN METAB-DRUGS	DOPAMINE NORADRENALINE	
ZINE CENT-DEPRESS-DRUGS	DOPAMINE NORADRENALI	
ORMAL UNRESTRAINED RATS	DOPAM	
ON CENT-STIM-DRUG BRAIN		
HYDROXY TRYPTOPHAN DOP		
T LEVALLORPHAN TARTP		
AMPHETAMINE		

ERASE/ N METHYLATION OF	DOPAMINE
D MORPHINE IN 6 HYDROXY	DOPAMINE
NCE 9-10 SEPTEMBER BOOK	DOPAMINE
ON OF A PERSISTENT HIGH	DOPAMINE
AND ITS RELATIONSHIP TO	DOPAMIN
NE ADRENALONE 6 HYDROXY	DOPAMIN
ACTIVITY NOREPINEPHRINE	DOPAMI
L P TYROSINE METAB-DRUG	DOPAMI
RIDOXINE ADMINISTRATION	DOPAMI
EROTONIN NOREPINEPHRINE	DOPAMI
AB-DRUGS NOREPINEPHRINE	DOPAMI
RAT PITUITARY 5 HYDROXY	DOPAMI
A METHYL DOPA HYDRAZINE	DOPAMI
NZAMINE AUTONOMIC-DRUGS	DOPAMI
TATIVE STUDY OF CENTRAL	DOPAMIN
KE IN NORADRENERGIC AND	DOPAMIN
-DRUGS/ ROLE OF CENTRAL	DOPAMIN
DRUGS MOUSE SARCOLYSINE	DOPAN E
HUMAN ALPHA METHYL DOPA	DOPEGI
TOGRAPHY UV/ STUDIES ON	DOPING
OMATOGRAPHY/ STUDIES ON	DOPING
GRAPHY A COMBINATION OF	DOPPLE
O VASC-DRUGS ULTRASONIC	DOPPLE
VASCULAR VELOCITIES BY	DOPPLE
VASCULAR VELOCITIES BY	DOPPLE
RING ARRHYTHMIAS IN MAN	DOPPLE
ILIZATION OF ULTRASOUND	DOPPLI
ITH TAKAYASUS ARTERITIS	DOPPLI
OF AN ULTRASONIC DEVICE	DOPPLE
OCRIT UPON THE SHIFT IN	DOPPLE
E A METHOD B METHOD AND	DOPPLE
UCTION HUMAN ULTRASONIC	DOPPLE
UMAN ANIMAL/ ULTRASONIC	DOPPLE
STAGE BY THE ULTRASONIC	DOPPLE
MENTS BY THE ULTRASONIC	DOPPLE
SC-DRUG RADIO TELEMETRY	DOPPLE
BITAL CENT-DEPRESS-DRUG	DOPPL
MAN ELECTRO CARDIOGRAM/	DOPP
ESSELS STUDIED WITH THE	DOP
ICAL APPLICATION OF THE	DO
TRANS CUTANEOUS METHOD	DC
CULAR GAS BUBBLES SHEEP	D
G MULTIPLE PREGNANCIES/	
OF THE VARIETY KNOWN AS	
H AND FRUCTIFICATION OF	
TRYOTRICHUM-PILULIFERUM	
ERATOPHYLLUS CATALLAGI/	
NOPTHALMUS-PSEUDAGYRTE	
AR AND ALTITUDE AUSTR	
ICISTURANII NEW SPECT	
RA FROM ANATOLIA TUR	
INE BIO ZONES HIPPA	
THE MARINE RESOURCE	
ICITIC SCHISTS OF	
IPERON NOLUDAR PE	
OTIC DRUGS GLUTE	
BILIS DENDRODOR	
GERMINATION RE	
D USSR FROST	
E GERMINATIO	
DRON-LAPPONI	
ORDIUM SUBE	
GATION AUT	
RA LIGHT	
SPONSE ST	
LIGHT SA	
AUCASU	
GLAD	
OR	

Figure 6. Part of a page from *Biological Abstracts* Subject Index, *B.A.S.I.C.*, Vol. 54, 1972, showing entries for dopamine. The underlined entry, for 62381, refers to a paper by K. Kuschinsky. "Morphine catalepsy in the rat: Relation to striatal dopamine metabolism." *Eur. J. Pharmacol.* *19*(1): 119-122, 1972.

AUTHORS' TERMINOLOGY
authors' terminology in the title. One must think of all synonyms and related terms for the subject in which he is interested. For instance, material on pediatrics might occur under "Infants," "Babies," "Child," or "Children" as well as possibly under "Growth," "Development," etc. To assist people in thinking of synonyms, BIOSIS has published *A Guide to the Vocabulary of Biological Literature* (BioSciences Information Service of *Biological Abstracts*, 2100 Arch Street, Philadelphia, Pennsylvania 19103, 1973. $12.00). It includes core-words that had been listed in the Subject Index (*B.A.S.I.C.*) at least 50 times up until 1968. For example, the core-word entries for "Cattle" and "Pediatric" read as follows:

CATTLE 11,443
see also BOS; BOVIDAE; BOVINE; BRAHMAN; BULL; COW; HARIANA; HEREFORD; HOLSTEIN; STEER

PEDIATRIC 1,942
see also BABY; CHILD; CHILDHOOD; INFANT; JUVENILE; YOUNG; PEDIATRICS-C

The numbers on the right are the frequency of occurrence in *B.A.S.I.C.* of the core-word and its variants — words with the same root and same general meaning — from September 1959 through December 1971. The "-C" following the word "Pediatrics" in the second entry refers to the CROSS Index to be discussed in the next paragraph.

CROSS INDEX
BIOSIS provides other search methods to supplement its permuted keyword index. One is based on the sections into which abstracts have been grouped in *Biological Abstracts* and other sections with which the editors would also put them if space were unlimited. It is called the CROSS (*Computer Rearrangement Of Subject Specialties*) Index. This is a type of presentation of index numbers which is vaguely related to bingo. It was first promoted in UNITERM indexing, a trademark invented by its early advocate, Mortimer Taube.[2] Under each of hundreds of section headings and subdivisions are arranged the abstract numbers appropriate in those particular places. In 1974 they began to be listed merely sequentially, but prior to that the computer placed them across the page in predictable positions on a grid, 0 through

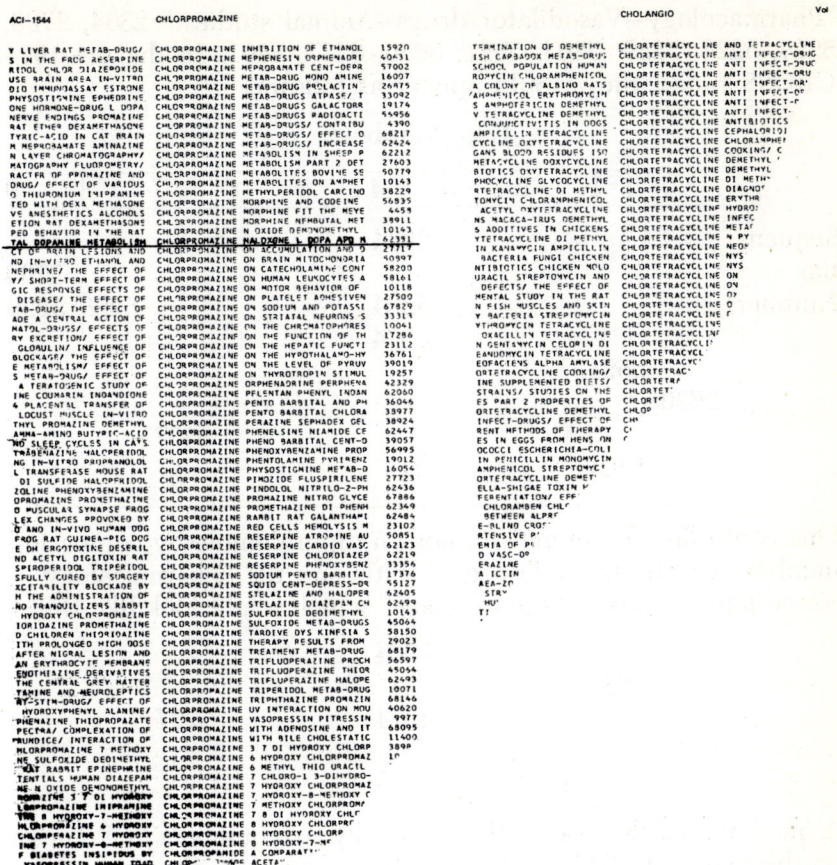

Figure 7. Part of a page from *Biological Abstracts* Subject Index, *B.A.S.I.C.*, Vol. 54, 1972, showing entries for chlorpromazine. The underlined entry, for 62381, refers to the same paper as that described in Figure 6.

"Pharmacology—Vasodilator drugs—Animal studies:" 2334, 2709, 5224, 5228, 5229, 5304, 5521, 5630, 8337, 8401. In the pre-1974 CROSS Index, they would appear as follows:

	End Numbers									
	0	1	2	3	4	5	6	7	8	9
Sequential Numbers					2334					
										2709
					5224				5228	5229
					5304					
		5521								
	5630									
								8337		
		8401								

One could find all animal studies on dipyridamole by comparing numbers on the preceding grid with one for "Pharmacology — Vasodilator agents — Dipyridamole" which might look like this:

0	1	2	3	4	5	6	7	8	9
				1204					
	2561								
				5224			5227		
5630									
		8402							

A quick match shows that there are only two numbers in common on the two grids, 5224 and 5630. Hence these are the two papers which discussed dipyridamole in animals.

The various aspects of the paper by K. Kuschinsky, "Morphine Catalepsy in the Rat: Relation to Striatal Dopamine Metabolism" (*Eur. J. Pharmacol.* 19(1):119-122, 1972, abstract no. 62381) were covered in the CROSS Index by:

Metabolism — Proteins, Peptides, Amino Acids
Pharmacology — Neuropharmacology
Nervous System — Pathology

Whether on a grid or sequential, the CROSS Index can be useful in correlating two or more broad subject fields and occasionally in coordinating a broad subject field with a specific term in another index, such as in finding neuropharmacologic studies of chlorpromazine.

TAXONOMY
INDEXES
Other indexes which BIOSIS provides to aid its users are the Biosystematic Index and the Cumulative Generic Index, the latter introduced in 1974. These have evolved from what was originally a taxonomic index to early volumes of *Biological Abstracts,* and they still retain some of the earlier characteristics. Taxonomy deals with identification, naming, and classification of organisms. In contrast with the earlier taxonomic index to *Biological Abstracts,* which lists genus and species, the Biosystematic Index does not list taxa below the order or family level. Instead, an abbreviated description of the type of study referred to leads one to the kind of paper he is looking for. Asterisks to identify new taxa are helpful. Specific organisms will be found in the Cumulated Generic Index to genus, genus-species and genus-species-varieties provided by authors in their abstracted papers. When the organism is included in the title, it also appears in the B.A.S.I.C. Index. Figure 8 shows the Biosystematic Index entry for the Kuschinsky paper already discussed.

In addition to listing entries for the Subject and CROSS Indexes, the *Guide to the Vocabulary of Biological Literature* provides cross references for the Biosystematic Index. Under "Rat," for example, one is referred to "Rattus" (the genus) and "Rodentiae" (the order), and under "Rattus," to "Muridae" (the family), all the information needed to check the Biosystematic Index. Obviously, this index is used most frequently in conjunction with others. For instance, it would enable one to find all the studies of chlorpromazine in rats quite quickly.

Besides providing its tapes to various organizations, BIOSIS has used them for in-house searches, on the basis of which they supply abstracts to questioners from all parts of the country. They also produce *Health Effects of Environmental Pollutants (HEEP),* which is included in the TOXLINE data base for on-line searching. Lockheed will distribute the services on-line.

Other Secondary Services in Biology

For the researcher in biology, two other sources will be useful: *International Abstracts of Biological Sciences* — which has a classified arrangement and for which the indexes appear very slowly — and *Berichte Physiologie, physiologische Chemie und Pharmakologie (formerly Berichte über die gesamte*

ACI—489

6791	RODENTIA	MURIDAE	PHARM NEURO	10089
·793	RODENTIA	MURIDAE	PHARM NEURO	10095
794	RODENTIA	MURIDAE	PHARM NEURO	10096
·95	RODENTIA	MURIDAE	PHARM NEURO	10098
?8	RODENTIA	MURIDAE	PHARM NEURO	10099
·9	RODENTIA	MURIDAE	PHARM NEURO	10100
·?	RODENTIA	MURIDAE	PHARM NEURO	10101
	RODENTIA	MURIDAE	PHARM NEURO	10104
	RODENTIA	MURIDAE	PHARM NEURO	10106
	RODENTIA	MURIDAE	PHARM NEURO	10113
	RODENTIA	MURIDAE	PHARM NEURO	10114
	RODENTIA	MURIDAE	PHARM NEURO	16007
	RODENTIA	MURIDAE	PHARM NEURO	16008
	RODENTIA	MURIDAE	PHARM NEURO	16009
	RODENTIA	MURIDAE	PHARM NEURO	16010
	?ODENTIA	MURIDAE	PHARM NEURO	16011
	DENTIA	MURIDAE	PHARM NEURO	16012
	NTIA	MURIDAE	PHARM NEURO	16013
	TIA	MURIDAE	PHARM NEURO	16015
	IA	MURIDAE	PHARM NEURO	16016
	IA	MURIDAE	PHARM NEURO	16019
	A	MURIDAE	PHARM NEURO	16021
	A	MURIDAE	PHARM NEURO	16023
		MURIDAE	PHARM NEURO	16024
		MURIDAE	PHARM NEURO	16029
		MURIDAE	PHARM NEURO	16030
		MURIDAE	PHARM NEURO	16032
		MURIDAE	PHARM NEURO	16033
		MURIDAE	PHARM NEURO	16035
		MURIDAE	PHARM NEURO	16037
		MURIDAE	PHARM NEURO	16038
		MURIDAE	PHARM NEURO	16039
		URIDAE	PHARM NEURO	21691
		RIDAE	PHARM NEURO	21692
		IDAE	PHARM NEURO	21695
		IDAE	PHARM NEURO	21696
		DAE	PHARM NEURO	21697
		DAE	PHARM NEURO	21700
		AE	PHARM NEURO	21701
		AE	PHARM NEURO	21703
		AE	PHARM NEURO	21704
		E	PHARM NEURO	21709
			PHARM NEURO	21714
			PHARM NEURO	21715
			PHARM NEURO	21716
			PHARM NEURO	21717
			PHARM NEURO	21721
			PHARM NEURO	21724
			PHARM NEURO	27690
			PHARM NEURO	27693
			HARM NEURO	27694
			HARM NEURO	27699
			ARM NEURO	27700
			ARM NEURO	27701
			ARM NEURO	27703
			ARM NEURO	27705
			ARM NEURO	27706
			ARM NEURO	27707
			RM NEURO	27708
			RM NEURO	27709
			M NEURO	27712
			NEURO	27713
			NEURO	27714
			NEURO	27717
			EURO	27719
			URO	27722
			RO	27723
			O	27724
				27725
				27726
				27727
				27731
				27733
				27736
				33271
				3274
				77

RODENTIA	MURIDAE	PHARM NEURO	39010
RODENTIA	MURIDAE	PHARM NEURO	39012
RODENTIA	MURIDAE	PHARM NEURO	39013
RODENTIA	MURIDAE	PHARM NEURO	39018
RODENTIA	MURIDAE	PHARM NEURO	39024
RODENTIA	MURIDAE	PHARM NEURO	39027
RODENTIA	MURIDAE	PHARM NEURO	39031
RODENTIA	MURIDAE	PHARM NEURO	45046
RODENTIA	MURIDAE	PHARM NEURO	45049
RODENTIA	MURIDAE	PHARM NEURO	45051
RODENTIA	MURIDAE	PHARM NEURO	45053
RODENTIA	MURIDAE	PHARM NEURO	45055
RODENTIA	MURIDAE	PHARM NEURO	45057
RODENTIA	MURIDAE	PHARM NEURO	45058
RODENTIA	MURIDAE	PHARM NEURO	45060
RODENTIA	MURIDAE	PHARM NEURO	45063
RODENTIA	MURIDAE	PHARM NEURO	45068
RODENTIA	MURIDAE	PHARM NEURO	45071
RODENTIA	MURIDAE	PHARM NEURO	45074
RODENTIA	MURIDAE	PHARM NEURO	45078
RODENTIA	MURIDAE	PHARM NEURO	45079
RODENTIA	MURIDAE	PHARM NEURO	45081
RODENTIA	MURIDAE	PHARM NEURO	50876
RODENTIA	MURIDAE	PHARM NEURO	50877
RODENTIA	MURIDAE	PHARM NEURO	50878
RODENTIA	MURIDAE	PHARM NEURO	50879
RODENTIA	MURIDAE	PHARM NEURO	50882
RODENTIA	MURIDAE	PHARM NEURO	50883
RODENTIA	MURIDAE	PHARM NEURO	50885
RODENTIA	MURIDAE	PHARM NEURO	50886
RODENTIA	MURIDAE	PHARM NEURO	50887
RODENTIA	MURIDAE	PHARM NEURO	50888
RODENTIA	MURIDAE	PHARM NEURO	50889
RODENTIA	MURIDAE	PHARM NEURO	50890
RODENTIA	MURIDAE	PHARM NEURO	50895
RODENTIA	MURIDAE	PHARM NEURO	50896
RODENTIA	MURIDAE	PHARM NEURO	50897
RODENTIA	MURIDAE	PHARM NEURO	50900
RODENTIA	MURIDAE	PHARM NEURO	50901
RODENTIA	MURIDAE	PHARM NEURO	50905
RODENTIA	MURIDAE	PHARM NEURO	50907
RODENTIA	MURIDAE	PHARM NEURO	50909
RODENTIA	MURIDAE	PHARM NEURO	50910
RODENTIA	MURIDAE	PHARM NEURO	50912
RODENTIA	MURIDAE	PHARM NEURO	50914
RODENTIA	MURIDAE	PHARM NEURO	50915
RODENTIA	MURIDAE	PHARM NEURO	50920
RODENTIA	MURIDAE	PHARM NEURO	56949
RODENTIA	MURIDAE	PHARM NEURO	56951
RODENTIA	MURIDAE	PHARM NEURO	56952
RODENTIA	MURIDAE	PHARM NEURO	56954
RODENTIA	MURIDAE	PHARM NEURO	56955
RODENTIA	MURIDAE	PHARM NEURO	56959
RODENTIA	MURIDAE	PHARM NEURO	56960
RODENTIA	MURIDAE	PHARM NEURO	56961
RODENTIA	MURIDAE	PHARM NEURO	56962
RODENTIA	MURIDAE	PHARM NEURO	56963
RODENTIA	MURIDAE	PHARM NEURO	56964
RODENTIA	MURIDAE	PHARM NEURO	56967
RODENTIA	MURIDAE	PHARM NEURO	56977
RODENTIA	MURIDAE	PHARM NEURO	62351
RODENTIA	MURIDAE	PHARM NEURO	62354
RODENTIA	MURIDAE	PHARM NEURO	62355
RODENTIA	MURIDAE	PHARM NEURO	62356
RODENTIA	MURIDAE	PHARM NEURO	62357
RODENTIA	MURIDAE	PHARM NEURO	62359
RODENTIA	MURIDAE	PHARM NEURO	62360
RODENTIA	MURIDAE	PHARM NEURO	62361
RODENTIA	MURIDAE	PHARM NEURO	62364
RODENTIA	MURIDAE	PHARM NEURO	62366
RODENTIA	MURIDAE	PHARM NEURO	62367
RODENTIA	MURIDAE	PHARM NEURO	62374
RODENTIA	MURIDAE	PHARM NEURO	62375
RODENTIA	MURIDAE	PHARM NEURO	62378
RODENTIA	MURIDAE	PHARM NEURO	62380
RODENTIA	MURIDAE	PHARM NEURO	62381
RODENTIA	MURIDAE	PHARM NEURO	62383
RODENTIA	MURIDAE	PHARM NEURO	62385
RODENTIA	MURIDAE	PHARM NEURO	62386
DENTIA	MURIDAE	ARM NEURO	6238[illegible]

Figure 8. Part of a page from *Biological Abstracts* Biosystematic Index, Vol. 54, 1972, showing the entry for the rat; referring to abstract No. 62381. (See Figures 6 and 7.)

Physiologie und experimentelle Pharmakologie (Berichte über die gesamte Biologie, Abt. B)) — a well-indexed, German-language source of abstracts to the world literature, including both books and periodical articles. Recently there have been a dozen volumes a year, each including 1,000-2,000 abstracts.

References

1. "Chemical Substance Index Introduction." *Chemical Abstracts* 76, Chemical Substance Index: 1I, June 30, 1972.

2. Taube, Mortimer, C. D. Gull and Irma S. Wachtel. "Unit Terms in Coordinate Indexing." *American Documentation* 3:37-46, 1952. (Also appears in Mortimer Taube and Associates. *Studies in Coordinate Indexing.* Documentation Incorporated, Washington, D.C., 1953.)

CHAPTER 14

OTHER SECONDARY SERVICES

Chapter 13 discussed the broad, general abstracting and indexing services of major importance to pharmacy and found in most large, specialized libraries. Chapter 14 covers several other groups of secondary services in somewhat less detail.

An Index with a Different Approach

Science Citation Index

First, there is a general science service which can be the source of choice for a given question because of its unique approach. *Science Citation Index,* like legal indexes, takes a key paper published some time ago and indicates all the subsequent articles that have cited it. In Figure 9, we see the references a person interested in drug interactions will find by looking at the citations to the work of J. J. Burns. For example, assume you know that Burns published an important early paper on mechanisms of drug interaction, "Enzyme Stimulation and Inhibition in the Metabolism of Drugs," in 1965 in the *Proceedings of the Royal Society of Medicine,* volume 58, page 955. You will find in Figure 9 that during 1972 there appeared ten papers which cited that of Burns, among them that by S. A. Kabins in the *Journal of the American Medical Association,* volume 219, page 206. From the Citation Index in which the above information

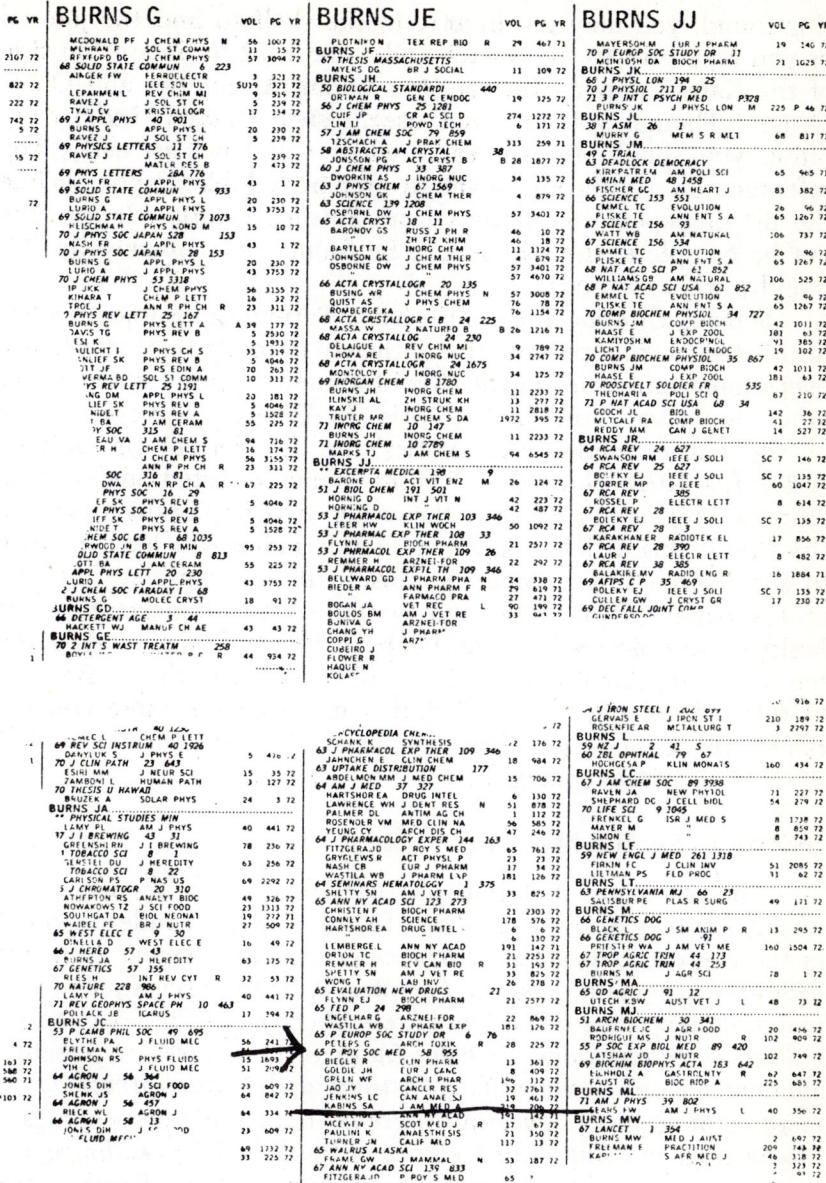

Figure 9. Part of a page from *Science Citation Index* 1972, Volume 1, Citation Index, showing the entries for J. J. Burns. The arrow indicates the paper which appeared in 1965 in the *Proceedings of the Royal Society of Medicine* 58: 955. All names indented under this entry are authors who cited this article during 1972, together with the exact citations.

was found, you may go directly to the shelf to find the journal or you may turn to the Source Index for 1972 to obtain the title of the Kabins paper, "Interactions among Antibiotics and Other Drugs." Though you may not use *Science Citation Index* very often, you should remember it when you have an early, key reference on a drug and want to prepare a bibliography. While the list of papers one obtains from *Science Citation Index* may not be complete, the papers can be found more quickly by this than by other methods.

Science Citation Index also has a Permuterm Subject Index, in this case a truly permuted — rather than rotated — index, since every important word in the title of a paper appears under every other important word in that title. In Figure 10, we see some of the entries under "Antibiotics" in the Permuterm Subject Index for 1972. Note that Kabins' name is listed under both "Interactions" and "Drugs," the other two important words in the title of his article. The user of this index will have to turn to the Source Index under Kabins to find a complete citation of his paper. If the title had contained ten important words besides "Antibiotics," the author's name would have appeared ten times in the reference list, under each of them. Because of this redundancy, you will find it easier to use more conventional subject indexes when you need to check the context of the terms you are looking for.

Indexes to Special Materials

Though many materials are excluded from the major secondary sources, they usually are found in special indexes. Some of these — e.g., *Dissertation Abstracts* and *Government Research Index* — are mentioned in Chapter 9, with discussion of the materials. To name but a few others, there are an index to translations — *Translations Register-Index;* and indexes to meeting announcements — *Scientific Meetings* and *World Meetings;* to meeting programs — *Current Programs;* to meeting proceedings — *Proceedings in Print* and *Directory of Published Proceedings;* and to papers included in meeting proceedings — *Medi-Kwok Index.*

Special Subjects

There is a myriad of special subject abstracting and indexing journals. We have named some of those developed as by-products

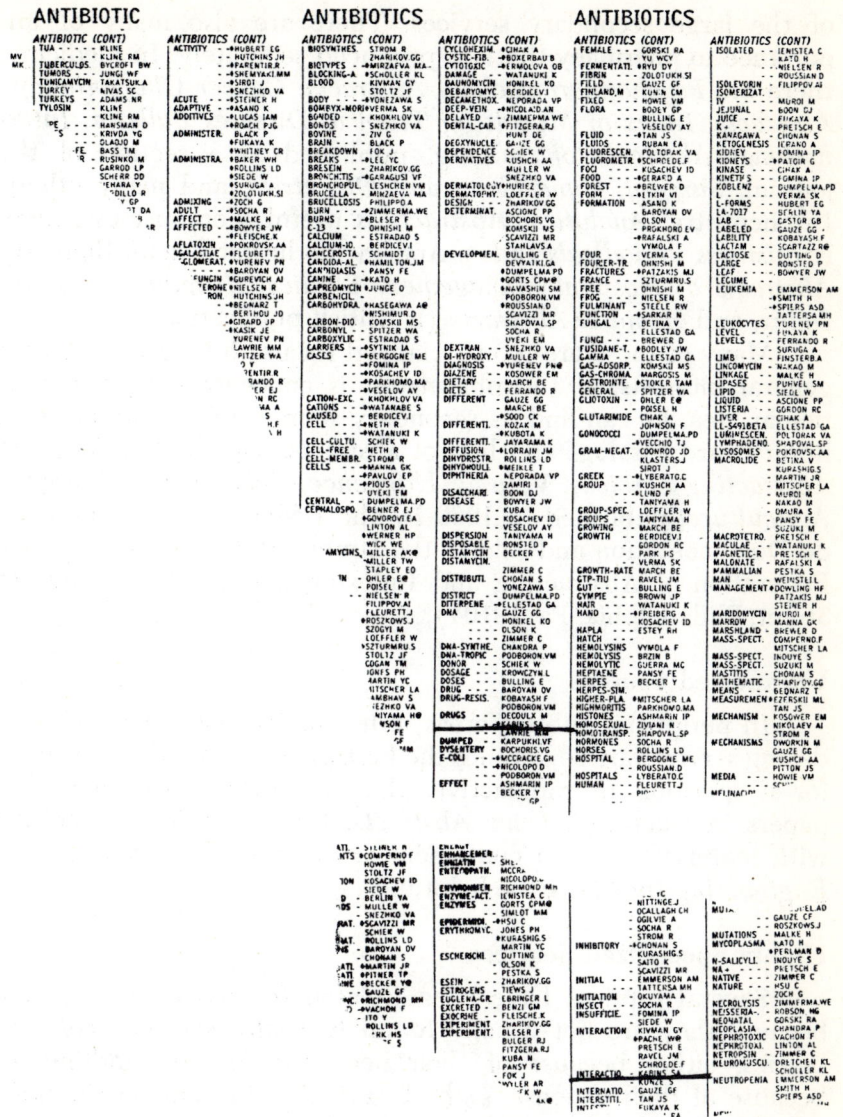

Figure 10. Part of a page from *Science Citation Index* 1972, Volume 7, Permuterm Subject Index, showing the entries for "Antibiotics." The underlined entries for Kabins under "Drugs" and "Interactio(ns)" tell us that we can find a title by Kabins in the Source Index which will contain the words "Antibiotics," "Drugs," and "Interactions."

of the large secondary services. There are also many of importance to pharmacy that are produced separately. In medicine, there are *Psychopharmacology Abstracts; Cancer Chemotherapy Abstracts; Index of Mycology; Tropical Diseases Bulletin; International Abstracts of Surgery*, published as a section of the journal, *Surgery, Gynecology and Obstetrics;* and many others. In chemistry, *Analytical Abstracts* is useful. For business, there is *Business Periodicals Index*. And in the hospital field, there are *Abstracts of Hospital Management Studies, Hospital Literature Index,* and *Hospital Abstracts* (a British publication).

Many of these are too specialized for use by the person with general interests. If the pharmacist is concentrating on a particular area, he can find its secondary sources by consulting local library card catalogs and lists of abstracts, such as the *Guide to Abstracting Services, Volume 1, Science, Technology, Medicine, Agriculture,* published in 1969 by the Fédération Internationale de Documentation and sold in the United States by the National Federation of Abstracting and Indexing Services (3401 Market Street, Philadelphia, Pa. 19104).

Unexpected Sources

In peripheral subject areas, other major abstracting and indexing services are sometimes the best place to look. For instance, for a question of radioactive pharmaceuticals, one may find papers in *Nuclear Science Abstracts*. For a problem concerned with materials used in containers or devices for administration, *Engineering Index* may be helpful.

Highly Specialized Services

Several services have been isolated for separate discussion because they are not usually found in health science center libraries, either because of their need for special handling, or because of their expense, or both. But they are among the most valuable in pharmacy. All contain abstracting or indexing on cards, and in most cases, the cards must be interfiled for the source to be of value.

FDA Clinical Experience Abstracts

One which can be used without card filing is *FDA Clinical Experience Abstracts*. It is on sheets that can be either torn into cards for interfiling or retained in bound form and used with an index to each volume. It contains conventional abstracts from a wide variety of sources, including some not covered by *Index Medicus* and other exhaustive services. All abstracts are selected because of their particular interest to the Food and Drug Administration, and hence their primary emphasis is on drugs in regular or investigational use in the United States. Each abstract has suggested index headings at the top.

The abstracts are distributed free of charge upon request by health professionals. Unfortunately, at the time of writing this book, publication is very slow and its future cannot be predicted.

de Haen Services

A group of highly specialized services is issued by Paul de Haen. Of greatest importance to the pharmacist concerned with clinical use of drugs is *Drugs in Use* and *Drugs in Combination*, a combined card service covering drugs actually being marketed, whether as single entities or in combination. This service is valuable primarily because of its effectiveness in scanning. The cards are set up so that the same sort of information can be found in approximately the same place on each card. For example, age and sex of individuals studied and dosage form and amount are included in the left-hand column. Adverse reactions are at the right or at the bottom of the middle column, depending on the purpose of the study. There are actually different kinds of cards for papers on therapeutic use and efficacy, clinical pharmacology, and toxicology. Each is arranged somewhat differently, based on the type of study, but the same kinds of information are usually in about the same place, so that one does not have to shift gears in thinking to move from one type of study to another. For instance, the center column may be called Diagnosis, Purpose, Reason for Use, Toxicology, or Clinical Pharmacology, depending on the type of study dealt with, and the third column may be headed Observations, Results, Clinical Laboratory Findings, or Therapy and Outcome. About 5,000 cards appear annually.

Drugs in Prospect cards cover the first announcement of a new entity and list twelve items of information: therapeutic, pharmacologic, and chemical classes; location of the study; molecular formula; nonproprietary and proprietary names and code numbers, if available; experimental design; inverted chemical name; and author, title and journal citation. There are some 2,000 cards each year.

Drugs in Research cards cover papers on a drug between its discovery and its marketing. A product information card includes the same general information as a *Drugs in Prospect* card, omitting the pharmacologic classification, but indicating previous citation of information on the drug in either *Drugs in Prospect* or *Drugs in Research*. The literature citation card contains a list of references in addition to generic name, pharmacologic and therapeutic class, and a de Haen drug code number. When a card is distributed, it may or may not be filled with citations. If it is not filled, references that appear subsequently are added to the old ones on a new card that replaces the previous one. About 2,500 citations are published annually.

The de Haen services are currently covering over 400 journals, about half in the English language. The cost of each of the services depends upon the type of subscriber and the number of card sets purchased, but if an academic library gets all services, the price will be around $2,000 a year. Another expenditure to be considered before purchase is the cost of filing. While it may take only one to one-and-a-half hours to file each set of cards as it is received, one must know that the filing will be kept up to date before subscribing to the service. For previous years, there are computerized indexes to the *Drugs in Use* and *Drugs in Prospect* services, as well as microfilm of the cards published.

Iowa Service

A hospital pharmacist, William Tester, has developed a somewhat similar service which also uses a computerized index, in this case as a means of publishing the cards and for local searches. Each card contains a reference and a few of approximately a hundred standardized "descriptors" indicating the kind of study that is involved on the particular drug or disease which are the key names used for filing. The unique feature of this service is that it also provides a microfiche copy of the original article. References are taken from about 150 domestic and 20 foreign journals, mostly with clinical orientation, and the data base now consists of around 25,000 articles published since 1966.

In 1974 all the cards were issued on microfiche to ease the

problem of filing by the subscribers. In two or three cases, experiments have been carried out with searching the files on-line.

Derwent Services (RingDoc and Others)

RingDoc, a service directed particularly to industry, has been provided for about a decade by Derwent of London. It was initiated as two separate cooperative services by European pharmaceutical firms, and includes intensive coverage of about 350 journals with research orientation, particularly in chemistry and pharmacology. It is marketed only to industry, since the basic cost is about $10,000 a year. It consists of good, detailed abstracts with structural information and tables, a "codeless scanning" card index to the abstracts that is almost an abstract in itself, and two computer tapes, one of a fragmentation and biological code index, and the other of the codeless scanning index. The detailed fragmentation code is useful in searching for drugs and chemicals and in studying possible relationships between chemical structure and biologic activity. The codeless scanning index uses a limited vocabulary, including some, but not all, of the drug terms found in the de Haen, Tester, and FDA services. Instead, certain structural features — such as "N-rings" and "S-rings" — are maintained as index terms. For each standardized term, there is a large card listing a half dozen or more references and several "free terms" describing each article in more detail. The cards are cumulated indefinitely and are available on microfilm. If one wishes to find all references to which two terms apply, it is relatively easy to take the cards for the two terms and see which sequential abstract numbers they have in common. Thus it is quite useful as a manual service, but its greatest value lies in the searches which can be performed on the computer tapes.

Derwent also supplies *FarmDoc,* an index to drug patents; *VetDoc,* for the veterinary literature; and *PestDoc,* for pesticide references.

CHAPTER 15

REVIEWS AND ENCYCLOPEDIC TREATISES

Even the most sophisticated secondary services are relatively complex and formidable. To provide short-cuts, scientists sometimes use the "snowball" method of searching, finding a recent pertinent paper, looking up all the references it cites, then in turn checking all the citations they contain, etc. For this method to be successful, the authors of the papers with which one begins must first have done a reasonably good literature search. An even more effective method is to find a recent review paper which exhaustively cites, summarizes and discusses articles on the general topic in which one is interested.

Review publications occur in practically every area with which the pharmacist is concerned. One has merely to look in the library catalog under titles beginning with such words as "Yearbook," "Annual Review," "Progress," "Recent Advances," or simply "Advances" to be aware of the variety which are available. They have in common the attempt to bring one up to date in a single general area. But they vary in methods of accomplishing the objective.

One series may review narrow subjects of current interest, including virtually everything that has ever been published on them. The subject scope is intensive, but the time scope is extensive. An example is the December 1971 *Pharmacological Reviews* (Volume 23) which is entirely on marihuana. With this type of review publication, new topics of current interest are reviewed in depth in each issue and they may not be covered again for ten years, if ever.

In the pharmaceutical field, other important examples of the long-range review series include *Annual Reviews of Pharmacology* (which also contains Chauncey Leake's "Review of Reviews" each year), *Annual Reviews of Biochemistry, Advances in Clinical Chemistry, Advances in Pharmacology and Chemotherapy, Progress in Drug Research,* and *Vitamins and Hormones*.

Another kind of review series limits its time coverage to the past year or so, but summarizes the activities of that year extensively. The *Year Book of Drug Therapy,* for example, selects all interesting papers and presents abstracts and critical comments on them. Instead of abstracting individual papers, other time-limited reviews digest a total subject every year or two and evaluate everything that has occurred since the last publication on the same topic. One of the most important reviews in pharmacy represents this treatment. The "Pharmaceutical Sciences — Literature Review of Pharmaceutics" article appears each year in the July issue of the *Journal of Pharmaceutical Sciences* and provides an overview of all the publications on a given subject in the previous year condensed into a few paragraphs together with a list of references. Though it has different authors in different years, the subject matter and organization remain much the same. Discussion is grouped into such broad areas as: general pharmacy, pharmaceutical aspects of specific kinds of drugs, and biopharmaceutics.

Whichever the approach, reviewing publications have become very popular in the past decade. They have the advantage that they can be subscribed to by individuals, and will substitute to a certain extent for the broader, general abstracting and indexing services.

Secondary services index review articles from many of the aforementioned review series as well as those which appear in regular journals. For those indexed in *Index Medicus,* there is also a separate *Bibliography of Medical Reviews*. For information on prochlorperazine, one would probably look only under that term in *Index Medicus,* but "Tranquilizing Agents" and "Phenothiazines" should also be checked in the *Bibliography of Medical Reviews,* since it is quite likely that some of the best surveys of prochlorperazine appear in the more general reviews.

All of the other abstracting and indexing services include reviews which should be given immediate priority when one is looking for papers on a particular subject, since they can shorten the search time considerably. A word of caution: if you decide to use a review, be sure you understand the ground rules under which it was prepared. Is it complete or is it selective? Is its purpose the same as yours, or is its primary interest research whereas yours is practice? And does it appear to be complete and accurate within its own concept? You may sometimes know of pertinent references, and checking to see if they are included will help you decide whether the whole review is reliable.

Related to reviews in function are the more extensive treatises or "Handbücher." While the German is usually translated as "handbooks," there is no relationship between these treatises on a field of knowledge and the drug handbooks discussed in the first section of this book. Any research pharmacist worth his salt should know about the *Handbook of Experimental Pharmacology* (originally the Heffter-Heubner *Handbuch der experimentellen Pharmakologie;* Springer-Verlag, 175 Fifth Avenue, New York, N. Y. 10010) which was started in 1920 and has claimed among its volumes such important contributions as A. J. Clark's *General Pharmacology* in 1937 (reprinted in 1970) and early basic discussions on the pharmacology and toxicology of metals and their compounds. In 1971, volume 28 of the new series, parts 1 and 2, was published under the editorship of B. B. Brodie and J. R. Gillette, with the title *Concepts in Biochemical Pharmacology*. In 1972, volume 30 was edited by Maynard B. Chenoweth and entitled *Modern Inhalation Anesthetics*. Though the publication was originally in German, many of the recent individual volumes are in English.

Another example of this type of publication is *Physiological Pharmacology, A Comprehensive Treatise* (Academic Press, 111 Fifth Ave., New York, N.Y. 10003). Edited by Walter S. Root and Frederick G. Hofman, this treatise projects ten volumes on various parts of the body (nervous system, blood and the cardiovascular system, respiration, the endocrine glands, etc.).

Finally, the *International Encyclopaedia of Pharmacology* (Pergamon Press, Inc., Maxwell House, Fairview Park, Elmsford, N. Y. 10523) is more similar to these comprehensive treatises than it is to what one usually thinks of as an encyclopedia. It is sponsored by the International Union of Pharmacology under the chairmanship of B. Uvnäs and contains such volumes as L. Lasagna's *Clinical Pharmacology* (1966, Section 6) and *Anticholinesterase Agents* (1970, Section 13), written by Alexander George Karczmar, E. Usdin, and J. H. Willis.

CHAPTER 16

RESOURCES BEYOND THE LOCAL LIBRARY

Sometimes the reference cited in a secondary service will not be held by the library you are using. Or it may be at the bindery or out on loan, but you need it sooner than the expected date of return. The first place to turn for missing journals is to individuals or to departments (in a hospital or medical school) which may have their own sets. Barring that, you must consider interlibrary loan, still a time-consuming process. The reference librarian will help as best he can if told when you need the publication.

Getting the Original Publication

When requesting an interlibrary loan, you may suspect that librarians have a conspiracy against you. There is a national interlibrary loan code which requires that certain minimum standards be met before the loan request is processed in a lending library. One requirement is that a source in which the citation was found also be cited. In library parlance, this is called "verification," and the requirement was established because so many inaccurate requests were received by lending libraries that their whole service was slowed in trying to find the article from incomplete clues.

If you have found the citation in a secondary service, you can speed your work (and make a friend of the reference librarian) by giving him the secondary reference as well as the primary one. If you are not sure of the accuracy of a citation, you may expedite the processing by checking the reference in the author index of the most likely indexing service for the year of its publication or the year immediately following.

Translations

A problem one may encounter in using secondary services is finding that the article of primary interest is in a foreign language. Don't despair until you have taken several steps. First, look at the original to see if there is an English translation or, more likely, a summary in English. If one is not available, check English-language abstracting services for an informative synopsis. If both of these steps prove futile, try to have pertinent passages translated verbally by someone who knows the language. Some libraries have translators on their staff or maintain a list of local translators.

Whether or not you have had passages translated verbally, you may wish a full translation. If possible, your librarian should check *Translations Register-Index* and journals which contain translations to see if the paper has already been translated. Custom translation, done for a specific need, is expensive, and not likely to be within the budget of an individual student or his library, but in some cases it may be the only alternative.

Networks and Computer Services

We have already indicated that a local library may turn to another library for publications which it does not hold. There are many other ways in which libraries support each other in their service to you, and indeed there is a network of medical libraries which may be called upon. You are most likely to be directly involved in using services outside the local ones if you need assistance in searching the literature.

The computerized abstracting and indexing services provide such help through one or more channels. In the first place, most of them issue lists of their publications and services and guides to their efficient use. In addition, customized alerting services are available on a continuing basis for those who have a need for being currently aware of a special topic. Or one-time questions can be answered.

There are three possible ways of receiving such services: through the regional medical library network, approached through one's local medical library; through commercial or university centers which maintain and process a number of computer data bases; or through the producers of the tapes. Whatever channel one uses, he may wait to receive the searches or, in many instances, he may obtain them directly by participating in the searching of the data base on-line through a remote terminal.

Since the situation is constantly changing, we will not list the details of the best way to approach each service, but instead suggest that when you have a problem you consult your local library or one of the national secondary services directly. They will be glad to recommend the most appropriate method. In order for you to understand the options, we will briefly describe the three channels and then discuss on-line services in general.

Regional Medical Library Network

During the past five to ten years, the National Library of Medicine has established eleven Regional Medical Libraries. They provide backup services to all other medical libraries in their geographic area and are in turn supported by the resources of the National Library of Medicine. They are concerned with medical library services of all kinds and, along with other centers, they did searches for their regions before on-line services became available. With the availability of MEDLINE, the regional centers still assist individual organizations in getting an identification number which allows access to MEDLINE or in obtaining individual searches from it.

Commercial or University Centers

There are a number of commercial or university centers. Some that have been in existence for several years are those at: the University of Georgia, Athens; Illinois Institute of Technology, Chicago; University of Pittsburgh; and Pharmaceutical Manufacturers Association Science Information Service, Washington, D. C., available to the pharmaceutical industry. Each of these maintains one or more tape data bases from the secondary services already described and keeps it up to date by periodic additions. Usually they perform both retrospective searches and current alerting searches. Even though more than one data base is covered for a single search request, searches are usually run separately on each because no two secondary sources are alike in the characteristics of the tape record, let alone the substance of the tape. It would be highly desirable to have the bibliographies combined, to avoid repetition of the same reference in the reports from several services. It is difficult to predict when this might occur.

Other commercial organizations provide access primarily to on-line services, and they will be discussed in the section covering that topic.

Individual Secondary Services

Most of the secondary source organizations make their tape services available to others as has already been indicated, but not all will provide direct answers to questions. Except for supplying registry numbers for chemicals, Chemical Abstracts Service presently refers individual requests to the commercial or university centers rather than attempting to supply customized services for individuals. On the other hand, BIOSIS not only makes its tapes available through the centers just described, but also provides customized current and retrospective searches itself. A feature of the searches from BIOSIS is that part of each one is done manually, assuring that completely irrelevant references will be omitted and that abstracts can be provided in addition to the computer printout. Not only does Institute for Scientific Information perform searches of its data bases on request, but it also has weekly alerting services called ASCATOPICS (ASCA standing for Automatic Subject Citation Alert) to which individuals or organizations may subscribe.

For other sources, one should write the publishers. If they are not prepared to do a search for you, they can suggest an alternative.

On-Line Services

The MEDLINE system operates under programs written by System Development Corporation (SDC) and named ORBIT. These same programs have been used by SDC to provide MEDLINE to Pharmaceutical Manufacturers Association users and others who do not receive it through the medical library network. In addition, there are other data bases distributed on-line through SDC, including CHEMCON (from *Chemical Abstracts*

Condensates), CAIN (from the National Agricultural Library's Cataloging and Indexing System), INFORM (produced by Abstracted Business Information), and ERIC (from the U.S. National Institute of Education's Educational Resources Information Center).

Another distributor of on-line services, Lockheed Information Retrieval Systems, uses DIALOG programs to make available data bases from the National Technical Information Service, *Psychological Abstracts,* and others, as well as the CAIN and ERIC sources already mentioned. As mentioned earlier, Informatics Inc. is making *Excerpta Medica* available for on-line search. They use RECON IV programs which are similar to DIALOG. Other data bases are expected to be marketed by these and other groups in the near future.

The National Library of Medicine is responsible for a second service, TOXLINE, which contains American Society of Hospital Pharmacists' *International Pharmaceutical Abstracts,* Chemical Abstracts Service's *Chemical-Biological Activities (CBAC),* BioSciences Information Service's *Health Effects of Environmental Pollutants (HEEP),* MEDLARS' *Toxicity Bibliography,* and Environmental Protection Agency's *Pesticides Abstracts (PESTAB),* formerly *Health Aspects of Pesticides Abstract Bulletin.* This service was formerly available on RECON programs which have also been used by the National Aeronautics and Space Administration and other government agencies.

Though the programs differ, there are many similarities. All are available for periods of about the last three years, but some extend further if the data bases were mechanized earlier. One gains access to them through a communications network accessible by regular telephone wires and requiring only a local call in major cities in the United States. The connection is made through the familiar telephone receiver that fits into a local computer terminal containing a keyboard which, with the exception of a few additions, is identical to that of a typewriter. Any one of a number of terminals which the local user may rent or purchase will communicate with all the systems. One identifies the system he wishes and supplies an individual code and/or password which insures entry to data bases by legitimate subscribers only. Each data base may be accessed by a number of users simultaneously through "time sharing."

To use each set of programs, one needs to learn between

a dozen and thirty conventions and commands which fall into five general categories:
1. A means of browsing in the vocabulary to find what terms are available — by using commands such as "Neighbor" or "Expand" to request a display of words preceding and following the ones you type.
2. A means of specifying search terms — by simply typing the keyword or by typing it preceded by some command such as "Select."
3. A means of using logic — requesting that both of two terms must be present in a paper for it to be retrieved (AND logic), that either one or the other must be present (OR logic), that certain words must not be present (NOT logic), or that specified numbers, e.g., for years, will provide maximum or minimum limits for the search (GREATER THAN or LESS THAN logic).
4. A means of displaying or printing resulting citations and abstracts in some instances — covered by such commands as "Print," "Display," "Type," or "Print Off-Line" (if one wants such a long list of citations that it would be uneconomical to use the terminal to produce it).
5. A means of signing on and off, moving from one subfile to another and requesting assistance ("Explain," "Help," etc.).

If one has used one company's programs for one data base, he can adapt quickly to that company's system with another data base. The systems can be operated by an individual with minimal training, the keyboard manipulation and commands being much less crucial than understanding the vocabulary and indexing conventions of the individual data bases.

All of the advantages of searching by computer are even more apparent when one does the searching on line. Whenever two major terms should both appear in a citation, it is much faster to coordinate them in a computer search than to look under one, the other, or both in a printed index. Computer data bases almost always cumulate several volumes of a corresponding printed source. In some cases, additional features not found in the published indexes are available in the computer. With MEDLARS, for example, there are added index terms as well as the ability to search hierarchically, using one number to represent many related index headings. Finally, with computer searching one has the dividend of a printed bibliography which avoids misspellings and other transcription errors and can be carried to the stacks for checking.

Where on-line services are available, it is always best for the questioner to participate in the search at the terminal. He can assist in establishing search criteria by guessing what terms are in the pertinent citations. Not all references in a data base that satisfy specified criteria are necessarily pertinent to the question; and not all pertinent references in the data base will necessarily satisfy the search criteria. If one is at the terminal as references are received in answer to a request, he can tell whether or not he is on the right track. With most systems, a list of indexing terms or the highlighting of words in an abstract make it possible to see why each reference was retrieved. Thus, with a little study one can ascertain what the "good" references have that the "bad" ones do not, and alter one's strategy accordingly. It is sometimes helpful initially to ask by author for references known to be pertinent and find clues in them for constructing a good strategy.

Costs

We have said very little about cost of any of the computer services. Because of the free public library tradition in the United States, people are not used to thinking of literature searches as having a price. All of the services discussed in this section do, although as taxpayers we have contributed to keeping minimal that for MEDLINE through the medical library network. At present many on-line services are being sold as a total package at around $50 an hour, exclusive of terminal and telephone charges. Many satisfactory searches can be run in fifteen to thirty minutes. For searches prepared at university or commercial centers or by the individual secondary service, one must be prepared to spend from a few dollars to as much as several hundred for a retrospective search and a hundred dollars a year or more for almost any current altering service.

One needs to revise one's thinking about the value of the search. He should realize that a great deal of time and effort is required of an individual to do a manual search. If preparing a bibliography from library secondary sources takes eight to ten hours, the cost of a retrospective search from whatever computer source might easily provide a net saving. If you choose to pay for a search, though, remember you are paying to avoid the drudgery of plowing through endless superfluous titles in an index to find pertinent ones. The more you are involved in the intellectual tasks of formulating the search strategy for the computer and deciding as to the relevance of the answers, the greater will be the value you receive!

CHAPTER **17**

PART 4

THE FUTURE

Some of us have watched the technology of information retrieval advance from a few applications of edge-notched punched cards immediately after World War II, through experimental use of massive, slow, nontransistorized computers, to development of the typewriter-like desktop terminal with a phone receiver cradled into it providing direct, instantaneous, English-language communication with millions of bits of information in a large computer data base. We know that there will be more significant advances in the near future.

On the other hand, the technology just described has as yet had little impact on the student's use of the literature and not much more on his professor's reading and searching habits. Even in industry and government, where many of the advances have been developed, the average research worker often is not fully conscious of the impact of technology on his ability to find information for research. Perhaps the greatest effect on today's student during his lifetime will result from technology already in existence. First let's see what developments affect him now, or are available whenever the economy will support mass utilization. Then let's look at what we can expect of technology in the future and its possible long-range effect on the individual practitioner. Finally, we will suggest ways in which today's student can take advantage of both the literature and the technology of the future to develop and hone his knowledge daily so that he will remain a truly professional pharmacist.

CHAPTER 18

CURRENT TECHNOLOGY

Before discussing technology, I should like to indulge in some generalizations. First, the situation is likely to get worse before it gets better. And second, there will be no real improvement until the delivery of health care information has met the same goals that the nation has set for the delivery of health care itself. There will be a multiplicity of different systems offered, many depending on individual gimmicks, before we find a truly superb system such as the "Memex" dreamed of by Vannevar Bush in 1945, where vast stores of information will essentially be at the fingertips of the scientist — "an enlarged intimate supplement to his memory."[1] The development will come in the future, as it has in the past, in fits and starts as inventions respond to real needs and as economics and social conditions make it possible to deliver information conveniently to its ultimate user.

Let's be a little more specific. During the development of information retrieval technology there have been several levels, just as there are in the development of a drug or a new kind of automobile. The levels of development in information retrieval technology correspond to the research, development, and marketing phases in better-known industries, but they are less clear-cut because the market is not so well established.

Parker and Dunn, in a recent issue of *Science,* pointed out that "the unit costs of public access to information could be reduced so much that the total expenditure on information services would probably increase substantially."[2] They talk of use of the computer to pair cable television with "subscriber response systems."[2] In other words, the student could call into his living room a videotape of lectures, slides, motion pictures or whatever is necessary for ideal learning conditions, and at the same time could ask questions or communicate answers to tests through a teletype-like terminal. The cost for transmission to the consumer of the needed information and data for "lifelong learning in the home" would be of the order of magnitude that we pay today for telephone service if there were a comparable amount of use. Parker and Dunn stress the need for a "regulatory means" of "nondiscriminatory access" to the system and also describe how private and public money would have to be invested in pilot projects to test an overall plan, but they conclude that, with proper implementation, the supply and demand could be economically matched.[2]

Computers

Turning from the economics of information handling to its technology, we may be surprised to find that computers already affect our daily use of information. Throughout our discussion of abstracting and indexing services, we mentioned such spin-offs of the main product as *Drug Interactions-1* and *-2* from *International Pharmaceutical Abstracts* and the *Toxicity Bibliography* from the MEDLARS production of *Index Medicus*. Once data have been put into the computer, they can be massaged and manipulated again and again into the forms and with the precision desired — always assuming that the information wanted was put into the computer in a recognizable and separately identifiable form to begin with. The abstracting and indexing services are natural users of the computer's capabilities because, like any machine, it performs repetitive functions well, and the function of a secondary service is to repeat or point to a single abstract or reference (the surrogate for the original paper), from all of the multiple points of view in which it might be needed. In other words, from a single input of a reference, a multiple output is possible. It may be entered in many places in a published index; it may appear in a number of different printed products; or it may be distributed to an individual as part of a retrospective or alerting search. The more often a reference can be used, the more economical becomes the effort expended in its original input.

The computer serves purposes in other parts of the information picture. Because it excels in analyzing masses of data in a variety of ways, it is used in scientific applications such as screening for new drugs, testing their toxicity, and collecting and analyzing data during their animal and clinical investigation. The computer has also revolutionized the printing industry because of its flexibility in organizing the data necessary for typesetting and in accepting last-minute instructions, changes, and corrections in final production. Thus many of our scientific journals and books are now produced by computer or will be in the near future.

At the other end of the spectrum, the computer is being used in the wholesale house, the large prescription pharmacy, and the hospital to handle inventory records, billing, and accounting, again because of its ability to process masses of material in different ways for different purposes. In hospitals, some patient records are also being computerized, and prescription records maintained in enough detail to relate the patient and his individual drug profile — again a task which boggles the mind of the human master but is cheerfully and efficiently performed by the idiot servant computer.

It is apparent that the computer intervenes at every step in a drug's history from its discovery through the testing and proving stage; to information published about it and its recording in secondary services; up to its ultimate consumption in dealing with a specific illness in an individual patient. It takes little imagination to guess that at some time the machine-readable data that are the output of one system will become the machine-readable data that are the input of another system, and we will have a complex of systems rather than many single free-standing ones, with consequent benefits in economics and feasibility for individualized use of the information, and with consequent hazards in possibilities for error and systems breakdown. One hazard has been increasingly discussed in computer-sociologic circles — that of invasion of individual privacy. We will not discuss this hazard here, but it is a moral concern of us all and may serve as a stumbling block to some of the advances we are predicting.

What we are concerned with is that the same technology

that is becoming necessary to move the drug from the producer to the consumer efficiently is that which is available to move information from the producer to the consumer. At some time in the future the margin between the two processes may become indistinguishable, and the information from the literature and the data collected in the hospital will be used in a single terminal transaction.

A word of caution: be sure you understand the difference between data and information, and then — for practical purposes — forget it. By "data" we mean single facts: the melting point of a compound or the readings from an electrocardiogram. When these facts are consolidated and analyzed, we have a body of "information." The term "data processing" was used in the past and is reasonably accurate at present because data is usually processed with respect to the drug. With respect to literature, it is references to information — not the information itself — which are usually processed. In future information processing, more and more of the original journal article can be available and manipulated in the computer, and more and more of the medical record or patient drug profile can be consolidated into drug information in the data base.

To summarize, today the computer impinges on every activity related to drug handling and information handling, from production to use. The individual pharmacist is probably most aware of it in his inventory and accounting functions since, whether or not he uses computers himself, his suppliers and third-party payers do. But today he is using publications and compilations from the computer. Both the *Red Book* and the *Blue Book* are now computer-generated. Each year some annual publications switch from traditional printing to computer production. In the recent past, this has usually meant a year of "agony and ecstasy" while everybody irons out the bugs and gets used to what can be expected from the computer. But, transition over, a new and better compilation results.

Input/Output Equipment

Tomorrow — whether that tomorrow is two years or twenty years away — the average pharmacist will be using today's technology, for instance the magnetic-tape typewriter, to process prescriptions so that he can supply needed information in different ways for different purposes from the same initial record. This typewriter is already commonly used in research organizations and publishing houses as well as in large commercial organizations. Or he may use an optical scanning device to read a prescription (in standard characters, not the typical physician's scrawl) which, like the output of the magnetic typewriter, can be translated to machine-readable data. It is difficult to tell which of these relatively simple methods of computer input will prevail ultimately if they do not coexist, or whether perhaps a newer and better method of input to newer and better computers will evolve before the technology comes into common use.

In addition to putting his own records into machine-processable form, the pharmacist will have direct access of some sort to one or several data bases which contain the records he needs to provide better delivery of the right drug to the right patient at the right time. At present one means for individualized access is a terminal such as those commonly used for on-line secondary services (Chapter 16). It is capable of receiving message through regular phone or wire services and translating them into meaningful keystrokes. Another means is a cathode-ray tube, like the television screen, which translates the same messages into symbols on the "scope." The advantage of the typewriter terminal is that a permanent recording of the message results, but the cathode-ray tube is better for transmitting diagrams and other non-print data and is usually faster than the terminal typewriter in terms of characters delivered per second. Another advantage of the cathode-ray tube is that a single tube can be seen by more than one person at a time for demonstrations, teaching, conferences, etc.

One's imagination can run riot as to possible applications. The physician could transmit the prescription in machine-readable form to the pharmacist, who could fill the prescription, at the same time using the information received to provide automatic labeling and additional instructions for the patient. While at the terminal he would check against the patient's current profile, review the recorded literature for possible contraindications or adverse effects, and use the record of the transaction for updating his inventory and for billing and accounting. The technology (or hardware) is already available. Some aspects of the systems analysis and development and program writing (software) have already been created in isolated instances or on an experimental basis. The question is when it will become socially and economically feasible to translate the technology into general practice.

You will note that in the preceding description of the prescription-filling transaction, I mentioned the literature in passing. This is as it should be. The pharmacist should be able to call on recorded knowledge in passing, indeed unconsciously. Only in this way can recorded knowledge truly have its fullest impact on practice in any field. Obviously this will not happen tomorrow, but it may happen in the lifetime of today's students.

Microphotography and Photographic Transmission

There are additional technological developments that affect processing of literature and other recorded information. One is microrecording. Microfilm has been used for some purpose for half a century now, and ever since its introduction we have been hearing that it was about to replace the book and other written records. It has come into its own very slowly as a substitute for scientific publications for two reasons. One is that there has never been a convenient, inexpensive, high-quality reader with which to retrieve the information once it has been put into microform. The other is that the amount of reduction and quality of reproduction have not been adequately standardized. Much work has been done on both these problems and it seems likely that solutions are imminent. A third problem, which can be solved rather easily once the major ones have been dispatched, is that of organizing and storing the microfilm, microfiche, or other microrecord.

There are basically two ways of organizing microrecords. One provides individual filmed pages or groups of pages on a card with a guide in readable print to what appears in reduced size. Depending on how they are produced, the cards are called microfiche, ultrafiche, microcards or micro-opaques, microfilm in jackets, or aperture cards. Whatever their form, the readable print information can be used to file them in the way most convenient for retrieval. Microfiche is familiar to pharmacists in the Iowa Drug Information System (Chapter 14) in which the drug and disease index cards refer to numbers of images on the microfiche of journal articles.

The other type of microrecord is microfilm in rolls, cartridges, or cassettes. Frequently there is a separate, printed index to numbers on the film which indicate individual images. The wanted film page can be located in a reader by devices to make possible automatic identification or by a rapid forward and backward movement of the reel until the proper image has been found visually. The automatic system is used frequently with parts catalogs and other large-volume, often-accessed information stores. It would be the answer to providing a massive drug compendium if the problem were only to bring all the data together in one place.

There have been experiments for years in communicating requested images of printed text across distance as wirephotos are sent. However, receipt on videotape at one's desk on a specific published paper from a remote library is still at least a decade off, even though experimental facilities are available at present.[3,4]

It now seems possible that the better solution to the problem may be to have locally stored microfilm linked to computer information retrieval systems. The pertinent citation could be located through on-line search in a remote computer data base, with provision for retrieval of the original article from one's own microrecord file.

Whether the new computer output microfilming process will have an effect on transmission and maintenance of the pharmacist's records is yet to be determined. Its initial use has been largely as a substitute for publication of bulky computer printouts because of the high speed with which computer messages can be projected on a cathode-ray tube and microphotographed.

As pharmacists know, many hospital records are already available on microfilm, which may also become the method of choice for storing a detailed drug profile, with only pertinent index elements being put into machine-readable form for computer processing. It is possible that at the same time analyses of drug adverse reactions at one's own hospital were being called for from a computer, one could retrieve literature citations and view full reports of both from the same microfilm system.

Audiovisual Resources

While we are exploring means of making the printed message available when and where it is needed, we must consider replacing it altogether when another medium better serves our purposes. It is well recognized that people differ in the ways they learn best and that all of their senses are potentially useful in receiving and retaining information. Craig has recently summarized strengths and weaknesses of audiovisual media for various applications, stressing the "illusion of life," "revelation of something new continually taking place," and provision of "a definite continuity of action" supplied by motion pictures and television.[5] Through animation, time-lapse photography, and slow-motion photography, the motion picture makes clear otherwise difficult subject matter. Slides have advantages such as excellence of image, ease of use and updating, and ready accessibility, and besides delivery of an oral message, audiotapes are convenient when one cannot read, for instance when he is driving a car.

Audiovisual resources can become a part of our routine formal and continuing education when their supply is economically matched with our demand as is already taking place with the tape player and recorder. In the meantime there is a variety of materials and techniques available which far outreaches the complexity and disorganization found in printed materials. Because the technology is developing and changing, the resources may become obsolete almost before anyone is aware of their existence, and consequently the means of learning of them are inadequate at the moment.

The pharmacist will discover a number of sources through his professional reading. The American Society of Hospital Pharmacists produces *Voices-12/60*, monthly cassette tape programs on various medical and pharmaceutical subjects. Like other associations, the American Pharmaceutical Association is currently distributing on cassette tapes selected annual meeting presentations of experts. The Pharmaceutical Manufacturers Association issues a catalog of films and publications of its member companies entitled *The Story of Health*. The American Association of Colleges of Pharmacy has a Committee on Audiovisual Education which has listed films, television tapes, and self-instructional materials.[6] Other pharmacy journals discuss audiovisual resources for self-instruction or for the lay public from time to time.[7,8]

Two individual sources for the physician are worth noting. One is the Network for Continuing Medical Education (15 Columbus Circle, New York, N.Y. 10023, with support from Roche Laboratories) which for a number of years has distributed new videotapes weekly for closed circuit television within hospitals. The other has been in use even longer. Biweekly, Audio Digest Foundation (1250 Glendale Ave., Glendale, Calif. 91205) distributes series of audiotape reels on various subjects such as ophthalmology, otorhinolaryngology, pediatrics, and psychiatry.

To discover the full extent of what is available, you will have to review directories of resources in public or university libraries, such as the Westinghouse Learning Corporation's *Learning Directory* (1970-1971), the National Medical Audiovisual Center's *Motion Picture and Videotape Catalog* (1973), the Armed Forces Institute of Pathology's *Catalog of Audio-Visual Aids* (1970), the American Medical Association's *Medical and Surgical Motion Pictures: A Catalog of Selected Films* (2nd ed., 1969), the University of Nebraska College of Medicine's *Preliminary 8 mm Film Project Report and Listing of 8 mm Films* (2nd ed., 1972), the American Dental Association's *Audiovisual Materials in Dentistry* (revised 1973), and the American College of Surgeons' *Motion Picture Library, 1971-1972.*

For a guide to equipment, there is *The Audio-Visual Equipment Directory* (1973-1974) put out by National Audio-Visual Association, Inc. (3150 Spring Street, Fairfax, Va. 22030, $10.00).

References

1. Bush, Vannevar. "As We May Think." *Atlantic Monthly* 176:101-108, July 1945.
2. Parker, Edwin B. and Donald A. Dunn. "Information Technology: Its Social Potential." *Science* 176:1392-1399, June 30, 1972.
3. Weil, B. H. "Document Access." *Journal of Chemical Documentation* 11:178-185, Aug. 1971.
4. "Full-Text Storage and Retrieval." In Massachusetts Institute of Technology. *Project Intrex. Semiannual Activity Report, 15 Sept. 1971.* Cambridge, Mass., pp. 94-95; *ibid.*, 15 Mar. 1971, pp. 46-49; *ibid.*, 15 Sept. 1970, pp. 73-75.
5. Craig, Robert S. "Overview of Strengths and Limitations of Audio-Visual Media." *American Journal of Pharmaceutical Education* 37:750-754, Dec. 1973.
6. Lowenthal, Werner. "Report of the Committee on Audiovisual Education." *American Journal of Pharmaceutical Education* 35:426-431, Aug. 1971.

7. Burkhart, Vincent de Paul and Peter P. Lamy. "Patient Education Using Audio-Visual Aids." *Hospital Formulary Management* 8:30-33, July 1973.

8. "National Poison Prevention Week, March 17-23, 1974. List of Materials — 1974." *Journal of the American Pharmaceutical Association* *NS14*:6-9, Jan. 1974.

CHAPTER 19

FUTURE TECHNOLOGY

You need not use a crystal ball to know that there will be inventions in electronics and optics that will create drastic changes in the equipment available for information handling — whether that information is collected locally or gleaned from the literature. As an amateur, I have been intrigued by holography — the use of laser beams to create three-dimensional images, and to store reflected light waves which can carry millions of bits of information in miniscule holograms.[1] In a gross oversimplification, one might say that such a device could replace the transistor, thus increasing by many times the amount of information which can be handled in a relatively small computer and thereby also decreasing processing time.

Holography could bring the courtship between the microphotography industry and the computer industry — which began with computer output microfilm — into a firm marriage, eliminating the division between searchability of references or other surrogates of information in the computer on the one hand, and availability of the full text in microform or in printed copy at a remote source, on the other.

When that happens, it may be economically possible to analyze and reanalyze the whole text of a paper in the computer. Use of thesauri, or vocabularies of index headings, as discussed in Chapter 12, would then become very different, since it would be possible to search for individual words used

175

in a text without any human intervention to index them on input. Many studies of text analysis in information retrieval have already been made, but they are hampered because of lack of sufficient data as well as by the novelty of approach. As these problems are solved, it may be necessary when one is searching the written manuscript, to think more about the author's vocabulary and language than about the vocabulary and language of the system. Eventually the system should be able to bring concepts together at the level of generality or specificity desired in a given instance, and the inquirer should be able to interact effectively to assure his finding everything in the system of importance to him.

A more difficult step, but one that will be possible with sufficient advance in linguistic analysis and increase in volume and speed of computer processing, will be the searching of literature in foreign languages, and their translation in at least a stylized sense, making it possible for the nonlinguist to understand the ideas of his foreign counterpart.

By the time this occurs, the price of today's television set should buy a home or office computer terminal that will link into any desired data base with no more trouble than switching TV channels or making phone calls across the country today.

There is little profit in a book such as this in going into further detail about the technology on the drawing board or in research. It has been mentioned only to indicate that we must be alert to radical changes that will occur in the next fifty years; anticipating them may help bring them sooner into our day-by-day life.

References

1. Leith, Emmett N. and Juris Upatnieks. "Photography by Laser." *Scientific American* 212:24-35, June 1965.

KEEPING UP WITH THE LITERATURE DURING TECHNOLOGICAL ADVANCES

The pharmacist has two reasons for keeping up with the literature. One is continuation of his own education to prevent early obsolescence; the other is improvement of his role as a dispenser of information as well as of drugs. Whether or not he is a drug information specialist,[1] he will need to answer questions on drugs, their actions and uses to maintain his professional status. The principles followed to keep up with the literature during the changes just discussed can be summarized in three words: organization, cooperation, and standardization. Organization depends primarily on the pharmacist himself — his methods of scanning current publications and maintaining records of what he wants to remember; cooperation calls for joint activities of pharmacists within professional organizations; and standardization requires coordination among national and international groups of physical and biological scientists and information handling technologists.

Organization

Keeping up with the literature requires both systematic methods of scanning and reading and convenient and efficient organization of what one wishes to remember and save.

During your academic career you have, or should have, learned good study habits and the ability to read or scan rapidly. One reads very few journals from cover to cover. Instead one scans the title page and turns to the body of the magazine only when an article of interest is listed there. One may thumb through those journals of primary interest, reading titles and abstracts of each article, but going further into the paper only if details are needed. There is another step short of reading the whole article word by word. One can read the introduction, illustrations, section headings, and discussion and conclusions of a paper and understand almost as much of its content as if one read it completely. Developing skill in all these techniques will help you to cover the selected literature efficiently.

In Chapter 7 we have suggested journals that you might wish to receive regularly. *Current Contents* and *International Pharmaceutical Abstracts* enable you to scan information from more journals than you actually receive. In addition, you will be buying reviews or up-to-date monographs that will digest periodicals you might otherwise not see. To find everything that is important, you should use your curiosity to discover new information in unexpected sources. When you go to the local library or to a pharmaceutical conference, make it a habit to look at new books. Keep alert to "what's new" even if your need to know is not apparent at the moment.

Much self-discipline will be required to get through the selected materials. Estimate how long it takes to review the number of journals you have decided to scan and then budget that amount of time into your schedule. All the organization, cooperation, and standardization in the world will not keep you informed unless you make a systematic effort yourself.

The ability to evaluate what you read will help you in efficient scanning and also in selecting what you may wish to keep for future reference. Before you graduate you should have learned the technique of evaluating the literature. David Burkholder[2] has stated the principles involved in drug evaluation by a drug information specialist as follows:
1. Recognition of the kinds of criteria in different disease states which might be measured in assessing the clinical outcome from drug use.
2. Knowledge of the natural history of the diseases under investigation.
3. Knowledge of pharmacologic mechanisms involved in attempts to modify etiology, pathogenesis, or symptoms.

4. Knowledge of all nonpharmacologic variables capable of modifying the disease state.
5. Familiarity with pertinent current drug literature.
6. Working knowledge of scientific methodology as applied to the clinical investigation.[2]

Many other papers in the conference on Drug Literature Evaluation at which Burkholder spoke may be of interest, particularly those on statistical studies by Hyman Menduke.[3,4]

Melmon and Smith[5] list the philosophy and salient features of clinical trials which one must understand to interpret current literature:
1. The purpose of the controlled clinical trial is the evaluation of efficacy and toxicity of drugs in man.
2. The guiding philosophy is the experimental rather than the observational approach.
3. The essence of such clinical trials is comparison.
4. The validity of the comparison depends on the accuracy and appropriateness of the measurements and on the elimination of bias.
5. The goal is to be able to generalize the findings to future patients, that is, to make inferences.
6. The strength of the inference depends on the validity of the comparison.[5]

The authors then specify the questions one should ask in reading a drug evaluation report.[5]
1. What is the objective of the investigator?
2. Are his methods appropriate and sensitive enough for the distinction he wishes to make?
3. Is the statistical design sound?
4. Do his data justify his conclusions?[5]

When all is said and done, the total of your five or six years of pharmacy training plus your subsequent experience provide your best basis for evaluating the scientific merit of what you read. If you have a complete understanding of the content, then it will be automatic to check for adequate controls, randomization of treatment, appropriate statistical analyses, and general objectivity in the assessment of therapeutic efficacy and potential toxicity of drugs. If you cannot relate what you are reading to what you already know, you will need to seek out basic texts or reviews to learn the necessary new facts and techniques.

Remembering what you have read may present a problem,

and inevitably you will be tempted to clip an article to keep after the journal has been discarded. *Current Contents* or a review publication may mention an article in a journal you don't see. For use in requesting reprints, *Current Contents* provides authors' addresses. For authors of articles found elsewhere, addresses are in directories such as *American Men and Women of Science* or *Who's Who in America*. Your librarian will be glad to help you locate them.

As you build up your collection of reprints, clippings, and pamphlets, you should be developing your plan for storing them so that they can be located later. Two simple methods of storing reprints depend on your memory. They are: to file alphabetically by the name of the journal from which the paper was taken and then chronologically within each journal; or to file by first author of the article and then chronologically within author. These methods have the advantage that they are simple and can be handled by a clerk. The disadvantage is that you will have to search in one of the secondary sources to find a reference to a reprint if you forget the author's name or the journal in which it appeared. If you have a relatively small collection, you can, of course, thumb through the whole file when necessary.

For a subject file, there are about as many systems as there are people who use them. It is wise to follow established nomenclature and classification such as that in a textbook table of contents or classification of a field, for example the *American Hospital Formulary Service*. If your purposes are varied, you may wish to use as guidelines the index terms in *International Pharmaceutical Abstracts* Semi-annual Index. Those building a more extensive system can consider major lists such as: *Medical Subject Headings* (National Library of Medicine, Part 2 of the January *Index Medicus*) or *A Guide to the Vocabulary of Biological Literature* (BioSciences Information Service of Biological Abstracts, 1973).

You might use a combination of one source for names for groups of drugs (*American Hospital Formulary Service*) and another for single drug names and other matters (*International Pharmaceutical Abstracts* Semi-annual Index). If you use more than one authority, be sure there is no conflict between them. To build your own authority list from scratch is an unnecessary duplication of effort unless you are involved in original research from unusual points of view.

The January 1961 issue of the *American Journal of Hospital Pharmacy* describes the Flack-King filing system for hospital pharmacy,[6] the *American Hospital Formulary Service* categories,[7] and a procedure for applying a classification in one's own organization.[8] For the individual, however, the suggestions of the Gaeke's may be adequate and quite effective.[9] They simply base their system on a textbook. Folders are numbered to correspond to chapter numbers and are arranged in a file box. The index to the textbook can support any cross references from one folder to another made by the individual. When interests become more specialized, the chapter numbers of a monograph in the specialty are used to expand the original classification. When introducing a second text, however, one must look for conflicts with the first and, if any are found, decide which text will have precedence in that area. For instance, if one decided to go into greater detail with infectious diseases, would the class of organism involved or the anatomic site affected be preferred for filing?

In addition to the subjects under which you file, materials and equipment used will require attention. Even though we have just discussed technology of the future, we have assumed that in the next few years it will be cheaper for you to file full-sized reprints manually and keep a minimal card index to refer to them. If you retain 2,000 or more separate articles and refer to them frequently from many points of view, you may want to create a more efficient index than the 3" x 5" or 4" x 6" card. Though it is possible to keep references to the papers in a computer, this would probably be uneconomical for such a small file. Other possibilities are mechanical systems such as "peek-a-boo" or edge-notched cards — both popular with research scientists and small information centers.

Edge-notched cards have holes around all four sides that can be clipped open to the edge so that the card will fall off a needle run through all the holes in a single position in a deck of cards. Since each hole is assigned a numeric, alphabetic, or coded meaning, when one wants all references that have that meaning, he can spindle the appropriate hole to drop only those reference cards that have been punched out in that position.

The "peek-a-boo" system operates in a similar way, but is

an "inverted file." Instead of a card for each reference, one has a large card for each subject term with a grid to denote numbered positions. References are numbered on a separate list. A paper's number is punched open on the grid card for each subject with which it deals. When one wishes to find all references on a complex topic, he places the cards for the appropriate terms on top of one another over a light source. Wherever there are holes with light coming through, he is seeing a position whose number represents a potentially pertinent reference.

One can summarize this discussion of building a reprint file with several precautions.

1. Plan ahead! You don't have to do a formal systems analysis to anticipate how much time is going to be available to you and your associates for filing material and refiling it after it has been used. You can also estimate how much material you will be adding per month and how often you will use it. What is the maximum size of reprints you will get? Can larger ones be folded to fit into the size of the file folders you have chosen? What subjects will you collect most about? In what way do requests arise — do they most often involve specific drugs, disease conditions, or procedures? Answers to the preceding questions can help you decide how your file should be organized. Remember the principle that the effort on input is inversely proportional to the effort on output. Rare use makes it more efficient to put more items into a single folder and do more searching at the time of retrieval from the system. Frequent use would justify many folders and consequent extra effort on input.

2. Make as many intelligent decisions on subject classification as possible in advance so that the day-to-day classifying of papers can be done quickly and a large part of the procedure handled by a clerk.

3. Use a minimum of different approaches. Many pharmacists can put the bulk of their papers under drugs — individual and groups. A file on hypertensive diseases may not be needed if there is one on antihypertensive agents. In fact, since most papers will cover both aspects — diseases and therapy — one should avoid the difficulty of deciding in which of two different places they belong.

4. Establish an authority list and stick to it as closely as possible. Modify it if you must, but do so with caution, exploring

carefully to make sure that the existing list has not anticipated your particular need and solved it in a way as useful to you as the one you are proposing.
5. Make the system easily expansible at the beginning. If you start with the *American Hospital Formulary Service* system, you might begin with major drug groups and plan to expand to more specific groups and to individual drugs. Or, if you are using textbook chapters, you might advance to chapter subdivisions or specialized texts in areas in which the file is growing fastest.
6. Avoid gadgetry for the sake of gadgetry. A punched-card or peek-a-boo system should be undertaken only after careful thought about all alternatives.
7. Keep it simple! The simpler it is, the more likely will you be to continue it and to use it.

Cooperation

To this point, we have reviewed the organized activities by which a pharmacist may keep up on new developments in his fields of interest, and retain information on them. He must do more if he wishes to assist in moving toward the Utopia in which the pertinent literature will be brought to his attention automatically as an integral part of his patient-care activities. In addition to his own organized approach to the problem, there is need for cooperation with others.

We have sketched elements of the system of the future, and we have indicated that these are not daydreams or systems being used in research only. Except for that mentioned under Future Technology, most of the technology discussed is actually in use somewhere right now. The problems are now those of making a socioeconomic transition from the technical capability to the actuality of having a computer terminal in every community pharmacy. One factor in the transition is the expression of the need through professional associations. After that, there must be agreement on standardization.

Pharmacists who work together or in close proximity can cooperate through journal clubs in which each member is responsible to summarize for his colleagues either important current developments on particular topics or all significant reports in certain journals. This is the first step in cooperation to extend one's literature coverage beyond what one can accomplish alone.

An important way to cooperate for a more complex purpose is to work through an already established association. We noted that the *U.S. Pharmacopeia* was initiated by a separate group, but that the *National Formulary* and *New and Nonofficial Remedies* were started within the already active American Pharmaceutical Association and the American Medical Association, respectively. All of the societies mentioned throughout this book have shown an interest in the drug literature generally as well as in specific kinds of information on drugs,[10,11] but perhaps the most comprehensive plan was proposed by the American Society of Hospital Pharmacists (ASHP).[12]

It considered the possibility of a government grant to support establishment of a drug information network, with about fifty regional drug information centers cooperating through an ASHP National Drug Information Service Center with the National Library of Medicine to obtain and evaluate information from the published literature and distribute it in forms immediately useful in patient care. Like other such ideas, this plan came somewhat before its time.

On the other hand, government funds made available in 1965 assisted in the development of library networks and regional drug information centers. Following the report of the President's (deBakey) Commission on Heart Disease, Cancer and Stroke,[13] funds were voted in October (Public Law 89-239) for the Regional Medical Program Project under which several regional drug information centers were established. The same deBakey report recommended strengthening of medical libraries and stimulated introduction of the Medical Library Assistance Act (Public Law 89-291, October 1965) which included provision for the medical library network. The Regional Medical Program grants were interesting in that they provided money for development of programs to support improved health care delivery, but the plans for use of the money came from the local areas, and even the organization of the region and the groups participating in the local Regional Medical Program varied depending on the individual situation. In a sense the Regional Medical Program and the Regional Medical Library Programs represented two exactly opposite approaches to the information problem. One planned and created a library network centrally (although local libraries applied to become regional centers). The other planned and created local solutions to local problems. In the case of medical libraries, many areas got library support through Regional Medical Programs and were then prepared to link their mechanisms for information dissemination in the region into the Regional Medical Library system as that developed. Though the future of the Regional Medical Programs is unclear, many of the activities they stimulated are continuing.

There are now several regional drug information centers and the number of individual centers serving single hospitals is increasing annually. While a medical library network has been created, however, there is no corresponding drug information network. Drug information centers, both local and regional, have cooperated on an informal basis and could begin to work together more formally — exchanging information and agreeing on certain areas of specialization for each — so that a broader network would be established gradually, whether under the aegis of a local organization, a national professional association, or the Food and Drug Administration.

Computers will inevitably be necessary to facilitate cooperation in a drug information network although it is hard to predict when and exactly how they will begin to be used. Several drug information centers use computers in limited ways for various purposes at present: for drug reaction and interaction monitoring; for analysis of patient drug profiles and drug usage in connection with hospital computerization or medical records; or for literature retrieval through a nearby terminal linked to Medline, TOXLINE, or other data bases.

More than once I have sat in a room with computer and systems people on one side saying, "Tell us what you want and we'll use our technical know-how to develop it," and scientists and practitioners on the other side saying, "Tell us what your general capabilities are and how much the relative costs are, and we'll tell you what we want in terms of how much we can afford." Usually it has not been said quite so clearly or simply, but that's the sum of it. There may be several hours of discussion, but frequently the two sides are not speaking the same language. This isn't too surprising when one realizes the problems in putting down the details of some of the grand schemes discussed earlier in this section. There are usually two or three possible methods of approach, and without having had experience with any of them, the individual pharmacist would scarcely know what to ask for, even if he had nothing else to consider. A great deal of time and effort is required for mutual education.

The problem becomes of far greater magnitude when several pharmacists or even a whole state association agree to work together to accomplish their ends. Yet it seems reasonably certain that the only way in which computer services will be generally available to individual community pharmacies will be through joint payment for developmental costs, computer access and maintenance, and other parts of the basic investment. Deciding how a network should operate to make his day-to-day practice most efficient is thus the task of the individual pharmacist working with his peers. To those who wish to determine the shape of their own future, it is an exciting challenge. Don't be afraid to dream, since without the dream you may never know what is possible.

Standardization

Though hospitals in the recent past have run independent computer systems, competitive with those of other hospitals, for some time there has been a general trend toward cooperation and centralization of certain functions so that now the exchange of records as a patient moves from one system to another is beginning to be accepted as practical.[14] Centralization of the hospital's medical record system with the aid of the computer began as early as 1955, when the Commission on Professional and Hospital Activities (from the American College of Physicians, American College of Surgeons, American Hospital Association, and Southeastern Michigan Hospital Council) began work on a Professional Activity Study (PAS), which provided computer services to their clients, individual hospitals. For the client, routine medical record data processing is provided, resulting in routine monthly, quarterly, and semiannual reports. Studies may be requested by the individual hospital, facilitating comparison with the general practice in other hospitals. Among others, the Blue Cross also provides data processing service to participating hospitals, but the systems are different. How it will be possible for the various groups to work together will have to be resolved. One key element of their cooperation will be standardization of the records maintained and of the format used.

One problem with standardization and with the development of a massive system of any kind is timing, since it is almost impossible to develop the whole system all at once. Should one part of it precede the other, or should two parts develop in parallel with no communication between the two? The latter is essentially what is happening at present with the systems of on-line availability of the literature on the one hand, and time-shared computer processing of hospital information on the other. The problem comes when such systems begin to standardize for their own purposes without taking into account the possible needs for linking to each other.

A classic example of the problem can be seen in the two present systems for coding drugs. Both are intended for use with computer processing and have inventory control as an important function. But one was initiated because of needs related to manufacturers and wholesalers, and the other was designed for the hospital formulary and management of drug distribution in hospitals. The *National Drug Code Directory* provides a unique code for every drug in the country with the manufacturer's designation being a key part of the code number. Within the manufacturer's code, the numbers used to identify aspirin manufactured by one company may be used for tetracycline under another manufacturer's code. While the *American Hospital Formulary Service* (AHFS) code provides a unique number for the manufacturer, that number is not an integral part of the code for the drug. The drug is coded to a generic name so that all of the drug products of a certain chemical composition can be brought together regardless of manufacturer. Fortunately, the AHFS tapes also carry the National Drug Codes for specific drug products, so that the computer can translate from one to the other if desired. In the printed *National Drug Code Directory*, like drugs are brought together in an Index of Established names.

To analyze a patient's profile to uncover possible duplication of a single compound prescribed under two different names or to identify adverse reactions or drug interactions, one must have information about the generic drug product, as found in the AHFS tapes. If manufacturers and wholesalers find the National Drug Code most convenient in their inventory control and billing, then both code systems are necessary because of the different purposes they serve. They represent standardization on two numbers rather than one. In a computer world, the dichotomy can be handled easily if it is needed and clearly understood.

The AHFS tapes are available for use in hospitals or elsewhere on subscription. Or the AHFS can prepare and maintain a formulary for an individual hospital from its tapes.

It is possible to solve most problems of competing codes and consequent overlapping networks but, until they are solved, there is delay in cooperation and the individual administrator must make complex decisions. Using an existing system saves a manager the time and expense of creating his own from scratch. In addition, if an organization just beginning to computerize — whether community pharmacy, pharmacy chain, hospital, or other institution — uses the same codes and data fields as others, that organization's information can be collected with that from other groups. Drug usage, costs, efficacy, interactions, etc. can be analyzed together to provide broader and deeper insights than possible within a single organization. It is thus important that the existing systems be made compatible with one another as soon as possible.

The problems just discussed with respect to computerization of drug information are similar to those in handling references to information in the literature. Because of the universal distribution of publications, problems of literature file standardization cross fields of knowledge and transcend national boundaries. The appropriate professional organizations and federal institutions have spent a great deal of time in studying requirements for standards and working toward their general adoption. On the other hand, a recent paper by Schipma *et al.*[15] demonstrates that much remains to be done practically. It describes the identification and file organization of the tapes presently available from different services. Not only are the intellectual parts of the records (such as terms used to index articles) different, but the actual methods of recording the information on the computer tapes differ in such a way that it is difficult or impossible to determine that a journal reference is identical in two systems. The recent introduction of an International Standard Serial Number should assist in solving this problem. An Association of Scientific Information Dissemination Centers (ASIDIC) has identified such problems in cooperation with the National Federation of Abstracting and Indexing Services (NAFAIS) and compatibility will be achieved in due course. For the present, the different secondary sources continue to be searched separately, even though a single person, using a single terminal and one telephone connection may move instantaneously from one data base to another. Standardization has been attained for the terminals and the telephone system even though it is not yet available for the secondary sources.

References

1. For a discussion of the drug information specialist, see Reilly, Mary Jo. "Special Areas of Drug Information and the Role of the Pharmacist." In *Drug Information: Literature Review of Needs, Resources, and Services.* DHEW Publication No. (HSM) 72-3013. U.S. Department of Health, Education and Welfare, Public Health Service, Health Services and Mental Health Administration, 5600 Fishers Lane, Rockville, Maryland 20852, March 1972. Pp. 69-73.

2. Burkholder, David F. "The Principals (!) Involved in Drug Evaluation." In Proceedings of the Institute on Drug Literature Evaluation, Philadelphia, Pa., March 11-15, 1968. American Society of Hospital Pharmacists, 4630 Montgomery Ave., Washington, D.C. 20014, 1969. Pp. 52-71.

3. Menduke, Hyman. "Statistical Design and Evaluation of Clinical Drug Investigations." In *Proceedings of the Institute on Drug Literature Evaluation, op. cit.* Pp. 100-113.

4. Menduke, Hyman. "Laboratory Session on Statistical Design and Evaluation." In *Proceedings of the Institute on Drug Literature Evaluation, op. cit.* Pp. 114-129.

5. Smith, William M. and Kenneth L. Melmon. "Drug Choice in Disease." In Melmon, Kenneth L. and Howard F. Morrelli, editors. *Clinical Pharmacology: Basic Principles in Therapeutics.* Macmillan Co., 866 Third Ave., New York, N.Y. 10022, 1972. P. 15.

6. King, Charles M., Jr. and Herbert L. Flack. "Classification and Filing System for Hospital Pharmacy." *American Journal of Hospital Pharmacy* 18:31-41, Jan. 1961.

7. Heller, William M. "Drug Information File Arranged According to AHFS Categories." *American Journal of Hospital Pharmacy* 18:42-44, Jan. 1961.

8. Jeffrey, Louis P. "Application of the Flack-King Filing System." *American Journal of Hospital Pharmacy* 18:46-48, Jan. 1961.

9. Gaeke, Richard F. and Mary Ellen B. Gaeke. "Filing Medical Literature; A Textbook-Integrated System." *Annals of Internal Medicine* 73:985-987, June 1973.

10. "Organized Groups Concerned with the Drug Literature." In National Library of Medicine. *Drug Literature.* Report prepared for the study of "Interagency Coordination in Drug Research and Regulation" by the Subcommittee on Reorganization and International Organizations of the Senate Committee on Government Operations. A Factual Survey on "The Nature and Magnitude of Drug Literature." U.S. Government Printing Office, Washington, D.C. 20402, 1963. Pp. 9-13.

11. Reilly, Mary Jo. "Providers of Drug Information Resources and Service. Professional Organizations." In *Drug Information: Literature Review of Needs, Resources, and Services, op. cit.* Pp. 32-60.

12. Reilly, Mary Jo. "Past Proposals for Partial Solution to the Drug Information Problem." In *Drug Information: Literature Review of Needs, Resources, and Services, op. cit.* Pp. 77-79.

13. The President's Commission on Heart Disease, Cancer and Stroke. *Report to the President. A National Program to Conquer Heart Disease, Cancer and Stroke.* U.S. Government Printing Office, Washington, D.C. 20402; Volume 1, Dec. 1964; Volume 2, Feb. 1965.

14. See, for example, Acheson, E. D. "Medical Record Linkage." *Methods of Information in Medicine* 8:1-6, Jan. 1969. There is also a bibliography of papers on this general subject: Wagner, G. and H. B. Newcombe. "Record Linkage; Its Methodology and Application in Medical Data Processing." *Methods of Information in Medicine* 9:121-138, Apr. 1970.

15. Schipma, Peter B., Martha E. Williams and Allan L. Shafton. "Comparison of Data Bases." *Journal of the American Society for Information Science* 22:326-332, Sept.-Oct. 1971.

CHAPTER 21

CONCLUSION

When the elements suggested — organization, cooperation, and standardization — have been put together, anything will be possible. This is not necessarily a message to each reader that he must show leadership in the three acitvities in order for the ideal to emerge. On the other hand, some of you will surely be involved before a useful system is available to everyone. In most successful cooperative efforts, we can identify one or two people who were determined to see the plan succeed. When these people appear, the mechanisms for success will follow.

As already indicated, in the very near future the resources through which one can get information from the literature are likely to be more complex than they have been in the past. One may have to increase his effort to keep up with the literature of his field and he may have to learn more about secondary sources than he would wish.

Gradually use of the literature will be simplified at each step. The creation by computer of tabular data summaries to include in journal articles and texts is possible as scientific information can be manipulated to organize and summarize test results. Standardization of the format of the whole journal paper has been suggested. While this might appear to hamper the author's creativity, organizing an article so that one could anticipate where he would find needed information would simplify the reader's task. Distribution of publications is likely to be routinized, with each of us automatically receiving microforms or reprints of all papers fitting into our defined "interest profile." Finally, retrieval of information or papers when needed will be possible instantaneously at a computer terminal or telephone or television set.

During the interim before the ideal, the pharmacist may feel he is becoming a systems analyst, and that standardization is limiting the kind of information he can obtain or disseminate. We hope that he will pass comfortably through the transition period to that where unit costs have been so reduced that he can build into his use of the literature those refinements that will be most effective for him. If we can get the right information to the right pharmacist at the right time, we will be well on our way to getting the right drug in the right dosage to the right patient.

INDEX

A, 36
Abbreviations tables, 11
Abstract numbers, 120-121
Abstracted Business Information, 160
Abstracts, 64-65, 108, 112-124, 133-143, 148-149, 151, 157-163
Abstracts of Hospital Management Studies, 148
Academy of Pharmaceutical Sciences, American Pharmaceutical Association, 68
Accepted Dental Therapeutics, 6-7, 8-9, 20-21, 29, 40
Acheson, E. D., 190
Acids, Latin names, 37
Acidum clofenamicum, 37
Acute Toxicities of Solids, Liquids and Gases to Laboratory Animals, 76
Adams, R. D., 80
Addresses, authors', 180
ADI, 6-7, 8-9, 20-21, 28, 32, 33, 39, 40
Adrenalin(e), 33
ADT, 6-7, 8-9, 20-21, 29, 40
Advances in Chemistry Series, 54
Advances in Clinical Chemistry, 153
Advances in Pharmacology and Chemotherapy, 153
Advances reviews, 152-154
Adverse reactions, 6-7, 7, 21, 27-28, 76-77
Adverse Reactions Titles, 134
Advertising, 25, 85-86
  book on, 69
  in periodicals, 60-61
AHA Guide to the Health Care Field, 93
AHFS, 6-7, 8-9, 16, 20-21, 27, 40, 180, 181, 183, 187-188
Alabama, University of, 48
Alcoholism, 88
Alerting services, 64-65, 157-158, 159, 163, 192
Alphabetic Categorized Lists, 128
Alphabetic List (*MeSH*), 125
AMA Drug Evaluations, 4, 6-7, 8-9, 16, 20-21, 23, 26-27, 40
AMA Seal of Acceptance, 26
AMA-DE, 4, 6-7, 8-9, 16, 20-21, 23, 26-27, 40
American Academy of Clinical Toxicology, 62
American Association of Clinical Chemists, 63, 82
American Association of Colleges of Pharmacy, 47, 51, 63, 172
American Chemical Society, 54-55, 63
American Chemical Society, Journal, 57
American College of Apothecaries, 61
American College of Physicians, 62, 186
American College of Surgeons, 173, 187
American Dental Association, 8, 40, 77, 173
American Dental Association, Journal, 9
American Disease. Origins of Narcotic Control, 78
American Drug Index, 6-7, 8-9, 20-21, 28, 32, 33, 39, 40
American Druggist, 8, 29, 40, 61, 92
American Druggist Blue Book, 6-7, 8-9, 19, 20-21, 29, 32, 33, 37, 38, 40, 168

American Hospital Association, 62, 94, 95, 187
American Hospital Formulary Service, 6-7, 8-9, 16, 20-21, 27, 40, 180, 181, 183, 187-188
American Institute of Biological Sciences, 55
American Institute of the History of Pharmacy, 63
American Journal of Clinical Pathology, 58
American Journal of Diseases of Children, 58
American Journal of Hospital Pharmacy, 59, 61, 64, 68, 90, 114, 181
American Journal of Medicine, 58
American Journal of Obstetrics and Gynecology, 58
American Journal of Pharmaceutical Education, 63, 68, 90, 93
American Journal of Physiology, 58
American Medical Association, 8, 12, 14, 25-26, 34, 42, 77, 173, 184
American Medical Association, Journal, 58, 62
American Men and Women of Science, 180
American Perfumer and Cosmetics, 62
American Pharmaceutical Association, 10, 12, 14, 15, 25, 34, 41, 63, 68, 70, 73, 76-77, 114-115, 172, 184
American Pharmaceutical Association, Journal, 61, 68, 93, 101
American Scientist, 61
American Society of Hospital Pharmacists, 8, 40, 47, 61, 77, 95, 160, 172, 184, 189
American Society of Hospital Pharmacists, Bulletin, 114
American Society of Pharmacognosy, 63
American Society for Pharmacology and Experimental Therapeutics, 62, 63
Amerson, Ann B., 50
Analytical Abstracts, 148
Analytical chemistry, 115, 148
Analytical pharmacy periodicals, 63
Analytical toxicology, 74, 75
Anatomy, Anthropology, Embryology and Histology (EM), 133
Anderson, Philip O., 73
Andrews, Theodora, 46, 86
Anesthesia and Analgesia, Current Researches, 58
Anesthesiology, 58
Anesthesiology (EM), 133
Anesthetics, 154
Animal toxicity, 6-7, 7, 76
Annals of Internal Medicine, 58, 62
Annual drug handbooks, 39
Annual reviews, 152-154
Annual Reviews of Biochemistry, 153
Annual Reviews of Pharmacology, 153
Antibiotics (Handbook of Toxicology), 76
Anticholinesterase Agents, 155
Antidotes, 6-7, 7, 74, 75
Anzlowar, B. R., 43
Aperture cards, 170
Apparatus, 15, 93, 173
Applied chemistry, 115
Applied Microbiology, 58
Approved names, 27, 33-34
Archives of Internal Medicine, 58
Arena, Jay M., 75
Armed Forces Institute of Pathology, 173
Aronow, Lewis, 71
Article arrangement in Subject Index (IM), 129
ASCATOPICS, 159
ASIDIC (Association of Scientific Information Dissemination Centers), 189
Assays and tests, 9, 10, 11, 13, 15
Assignees, 87
Association of Scientific Information Dissemination Centers (ASIDIC), 189
Associations, pharmaceutical, 93, 177, 184, 186
Atomic weights, 11
Audio Digest Foundation, 173

INDEX

Audiotapes, 172, 173
Audio-Visual Equipment Directory, 173
Audiovisual Materials in Dentistry, 173
Audiovisual resources, 78-79, 172-173
Author Index (CA), 115
Authority of drug handbooks, 8, 10, 12, 14, 24-28
Authority lists, 109, 116-118, 125, 151
Authors' addresses, 180
Author's terminology (natural language), 109, 138-139, 151, 176
Automatic Subject Citation Alert (ASCA), 159
Automedication, 31
Availability, market, 6, 6-7
Aviado, Domingo M., 71

Ba, 36
Backwards cross references, 126-127
Baker, Charles E., Jr., 42
Baker, S. B. de C., 68
B.A.S.I.C., 135-138
"Basic Journal List for Small Hospital Libraries," 52
Beeson, Paul B., 80
Bell, J. Edward, 83
Bennett, I. L., 80
Berichte über die gesamte Biologie, 143
Berichte über die gesamte Physiologie und experimentelle Pharmakologie, 143
Berichte Physiologie, physiologische Chemie und Pharmakologie, 143
Berton, Alberta D., 86
"Best Sources of Drug-Therapy Information," 46
Best & Taylor's Physiological Basis of Medical Practice, 79
Bibliographies, 6-7, 18, 46-55, 85, 88, 114, 132, 153
Bibliographies, biology, 54-55
Bibliographies, chemistry, 54-55
Bibliographies, medical, 52-53, 132, 153

"Bibliography of Books and Reference Works Relating to the Professional Courses in the Pharmaceutical Curriculum," 50, 70
Bibliography of Medical Reviews, 153-154
Bibliography of Pharmaceutical Reference Literature, 48
Biglieri, Edward G., 80
Biochemical and Biophysical Research Communications, 58, 59
Biochemical Pharmacology, 62
Biochemistry, 81-83, 115
Biological Abstracts, 124, 135-143
Biological and Biomedical Resource Literature, 54
Biological Sciences (Directory of Information Resources in the United States), 90
Biologicals, veterinary, 14, 22
Biology bibliographies, 54-55
Biology secondary publications, 135-143
Biopharmaceutics, 70, 72
"Biopharmaceutics" (Literature review), 72
Biopharmaceutics and Pharmacokinetics; An Introduction, 72
Biopharmaceutics and Relevant Pharmacokinetics, 72
Bioresearch Index, 135
BioScience, 61
Biosciences Information Service of *Biological Abstracts* (BIOSIS), 135-143, 159, 160, 180
BIOSIS (Biosciences Information Service of *Biological Abstracts*), 135-143, 159, 160, 180
Biosystematic Index (BIOSIS), 141-143
Blacow, Norman W., 40
Blakiston's New Gould Medical Dictionary, 79
Blissitt, Charles W., 51, 73
Block, Seymour S., 69
Bloomfield, J. C., 28, 46
Blue Book, 6-7, 8-9, 19, 20-21, 29, 32,

33, 37, 38, 40, 168
Blue Book, Veterinarian's, 6-7, 14-15, 22-23, 29, 43
Blue Cross, 187
"Blue Sheet," 62
Bonnett, Howard T., 55
Book catalogs, library, 98, 101-103
Book reviews, 15, 58, 68
Books, 67-83, 98
Books, chemistry, 81-83, 121
Books, medicine, 79-81
Books, pharmacology, 70-73
Books, pharmacy, 68-70
Books, toxicology, 74-77
"Books for Pharmacy Colleges," 46, 70
Botanicals, 9
Bottle, R. T., 54, 55
Bourne, Peter G., 78
Bower, C. A., 66
Bradley, Willis T., 69
Brady, Lynn R., 69
Brandon, Alfred N., 52, 80, 81, 82
Braunwald, E., 80
Breeding chart, 15
British drugs, 28
British Journal of Anaesthesia, 58
British Journal of Pharmacology, 62
British Medical Association, 62
British Medical Journal, 62
British National Formulary, 28
British Pharmaceutical Codex, 28
British Pharmacological Society, 62
British Pharmacopoeia, 28, 33
British Veterinary Codex, 28
Brobeck, John R., 79
Brodie, B. B., 154
Brown, Thomas R., 95
Brunn, Alice Lefler, 46
"Building a Clinically-Oriented Drug Information Service," 46
Bulletin of the American Society of Hospital Pharmacists, 114
Bulletin of the Trademark Bureau of the PMA, 35
Burger, Alfred, 82
Burkhart, Vincent de Paul, 174
Burkholder, David F., 179, 189

Burman, C. R., 54
Burns, J. J., 144-145
Burroughs Wellcome, 36
Bush, Vannevar, 165, 173
Business operations, 85, 115
Business Periodicals Index, 148
BW, 36

CA Condensates, 116, 122, 160
CA Integrated Subject File, 122
CA Subject Index Alert, 122
Cable television, 166
CAIN, 160
California Medicine, 60, 98
Canadian Compendium of Pharmaceutical Specialties, 6-7, 8-9, 20-21, 40
Canadian drugs, 8-9, 11, 13, 17
Canadian Journal of Hospital Pharmacy, 61
Canadian Medical Association Journal, 21
Canadian Pharmaceutical Association, 8, 40, 61
Canadian Pharmaceutical Journal, 21, 61
Canadian regulations, 9
Canadian Society of Hospital Pharmacists, 61
Cancer Chemotherapy Abstracts, 148
Cancer Chemotherapy Reports, 58
Cancer Research, 58
Card catalog, library, 98, 101-103
Card files, 44, 102-103
Card services, 39, 44, 74, 148-151
Cardiovascular Diseases and Cardiovascular Surgery (EM), 133
Cards, edge-notched, 181-182
Cards, peek-a-boo, 181-182
Carr, C. Jelleff, 71
Cartridges, microfilm, 171
CAS numbers, 15, 23, 89, 122
Cassettes, microfilm, 171
Catalog, library, 98, 101-103
Catalog of Audio-Visual Aids, 173
Catalog cards, 102-103
Categorized Lists (*MeSH*), 125, 127
Categorized Lists, Alphabetic, 128

Cathode ray tube terminals, 169
Catholic Hospital Association, 62
CBAC (Chemical-Biological Activities), 122, 160
CBE Style Manual, 54
Cecil-Loeb Textbook of Medicine, 80
Central Society for Clinical Research, 63
Centre Scientifique de la Société de Pharmacie, 41
Cerebrovascular Bibliography, 132
Chain drug industry, 92
Chain Store Age, 61, 92
Change principle in searching, 110
Changes in *Medical Subject Headings*, 128
Chatton, Milton J., 79, 80
Check tags, 131
CHEMCON, 160
Chemical Abstracts, 35, 87, 114, 115-123
Chemical Abstracts Service, 89, 117-118, 159, 160
Chemical Abstracts Information Services, 122
Chemical-Biological Activities (*CBAC*), 122, 160
Chemical-biological activity correlation, 151
Chemical engineering, 115
Chemical and Engineering News, 57
Chemical entities, 9, 11, 13, 31-32, 119-120
Chemical groups (fragments, substructures), 23, 122, 124, 151
Chemical index arrangement, 118-119
Chemical names, 13, 35, 89
Chemical nomenclature, 35, 117-118
Chemical periodicals, 54-55, 57-58, 62-63, 65
Chemical properties, 6-7, 17, 75, 95
Chemical Publications. Their Nature and Use, 54, 82, 87
Chemical reactions, 13, 124
Chemical Reviews, 57
Chemical rings, 13, 121-122
Chemical searching in BIOSIS, 136-138
Chemical searching in *Index Medicus*, 129-131
Chemical Substance Index (*CA*), 116-120, 143
Chemical Substructure Index; Structure Index to Current Abstracts of Chemistry and Index Chemicus, 124
Chemical Week, 57
Chemistry, analytical, 115, 148
Chemistry, applied, 115
Chemistry, clinical, 63, 82-83, 95
Chemistry, inorganic, 81-83
Chemistry, macromolecular, 115
Chemistry, medicinal, 46, 54-55, 82
Chemistry, organic, 81-83, 115, 151
Chemistry, physical, 115
Chemistry bibliographies, 54-55
Chemistry books, 81-83, 121
Chemistry of Industrial Toxicology, 75
Chemistry and Industry, 57
Chemistry secondary publications, 115-124
Chenoweth, Maynard B., 154
Choosing a personal collection, 6-7, 38-44, 50, 64-65, 67-68, 85-86, 88, 153, 178-183
Ciba Geigy Journal, 84
CIBA Pharmaceutical Company, 36, 84
Citation Index (*SCI*), 145-146
Citation searches, 109, 144-147, 152
Citation studies, 64
Claims, patent, 86
Clark, A. J., 154
Clarke, E. G. C., 7, 30, 41, 75
Classification of organisms, 141-143
Classifications, library, 99-101
Claus, Edward P., 69
Clearinghouse Announcements in Science and Technology, 89
ClinAlert, 65, 76
Clinical chemistry, 63, 82-83, 95
Clinical Chemistry, 63
Clinical Diagnosis by Laboratory Methods, 82
Clinical Interpretation of Laboratory Tests, 82
Clinical Laboratory Diagnosis, 82

Clinical Pediatrics, 62
Clinical pharmacology, 70, 73
Clinical Pharmacology, 155
Clinical Pharmacology; Basic Principles in Therapeutics, 73
Clinical Pharmacology and Therapeutics, 62
Clinical pharmacy, 70, 73
Clinical pharmacy periodicals, 62
Clinical Pharmacy Practice, 51, 73
Clinical Pharmacy Services in a Community Hospital, 73
Clinical Toxicology, 62
Clinical Toxicology of Commercial Products, 74
Clinical trials, 179
See also Investigational drugs
Clofenamic acid, Latin name, 37
Closed circuit television, 173
Code of Federal Regulations, Title 21, 27
Code numbers, 13, 15, 22, 23, 30, 36, 187-188
Codeless scanning, 151
Coleman, James S., 91
Coleman, Thomas E., 69
Colleagues as information source, 97
Collecting a personal library, 6-7, 38-44, 50, 64-65, 67-68, 85-86, 88, 153, 178-183
Colleges of pharmacy, 46, 50, 70, 93
Colors, 89
Combinations, 9, 11, 15, 31-32
Commands, computer, 161
Commercial products, 74
Commercial search services, 158-159
Commission on Professional and Hospital Activities, 186-187
Committee on Audiovisual Education, AACP, 172
Common names, 34, 35
Communication networks, 160-161, 169
Community pharmacy, 69, 85, 92, 93, 115, 167, 188
Community pharmacy periodicals, 61
Comparative Guide of Veterinary and Human Pharmaceuticals, 15
Comparative prices, 7, 10-11, 29

Comparison of products, 10-11
Compendium, universal, 4-5, 171
Compendium of Pharmaceutical Specialties, 6-7, 8-9, 20-21, 40
"Comprehensive Bibliography on Hospital Pharmacy," 114
Computer output microfilm, 171, 175
Computer Rearrangement of Subject Specialties (CROSS) Index, 139-141
Computer systems, 93, 113, 157-163, 166-168, 181, 185
See also On-line services
Computer tapes, 113, 114, 122, 124, 131-132, 134, 143, 151, 159, 188, 189
Computer terminals, 160-161, 169, 176, 185, 192
Concepts in Biochemical Pharmacology, 154
Conference on Drug Literature Evaluation, 179
Congressional hearings, 88
Constantino, Norma V., 83
Consumer newsletters, 64
Consumers, 70, 173
Containers, 93, 148
Contents lists, 64-65, 178
Continuing education, 166, 172, 177
Contraceptives, oral, 32
Contraindications, 6-7, 7
See also Therapeutic incompatibilities
Conversion tables, 9
Cooperation, 177, 183-186, 191
COPNIP List, 86
Cosmetics, 47, 62, 63, 89
Cost of drugs, 6, 6-7, 29
Cost of handbooks, 40-43, 44
Cost of searches, 162-163, 165-166
Council of Biology Editors, Committee on Form and Style, 54
Council on Dental Therapeutics, 8
Council on Drugs, American Medical Association, 12, 25, 26
Council of Pharmaceutical Society of Great Britain, 10
Council on Pharmacy and Chemistry, American Medical Association, 25

CPS, 6-7, 8-9, 20-21, 40
Craig, Robert S., 172, 174
CRC Manual of Analytical Toxicology, 75
Credit information, 93
CROSS (Computer Rearrangement of Subject Specialties) Index, 139-141
Cross references (*MeSH*), 125-127
CRT terminals, 169
Cumulated Generic Index (BIOSIS), 141
Cumulated Index Medicus, 110, 113, 114, 125-133, 134, 149, 153, 166, 180
Cumulated indexes (*CA*), 116
Cumulated list of changes (*MeSH*), 128
Cumulated List of New Medical Subject Headings 1963-1973, 110, 128
Current Abstracts of Chemistry and Index Chemicus, 124
Current alerting services, 64-65, 157-158, 159, 163, 192
Current Concepts in the Pharmaceutical Sciences: Dosage Form Design and Bioavailability, 72
Current Contents, 65, 124, 178, 180
Current Contents/Clinical Practice, 65
Current Contents/Life Sciences, 65
Current Contents/Physical and Chemical Sciences, 65
Current Contents/Social and Behavioral Sciences, 65
Current Drug Handbook, 6-7, 8-9, 20-21, 29, 40
Current Medical Diagnosis and Treatment, 79
Current Programs, 146
Current Researches, Anesthesia and Analgesia, 58
Current technology, 165-174
Current Therapeutic Research, 60
Curry, Alan S., 75
Curry, Stephen H., 72
Customer newsletters, 64
Customers, 70, 173
Customized searches, 114, 143, 157-158, 159, 162-163
Cutting, Windsor C., 71

Cyclic AMP, 85

Dangerous Properties of Industrial Materials, 74
Data processing, 168
Data Sheets (Manufacturing Chemist's Association), 74
Date of first announcement of drugs, 6-7, 149-150
Date of introduction, 9, 13, 17, 87, 109
Date of issuance of patents, 87, 109
Davidsohn, Israel, 82
Davis, Bernard D., 81
Deans, colleges of pharmacy, 93
deBakey report, 184-185
Definitions of subject headings, 126-128
deHaen, Paul, 6-7, 8, 20, 40, 46, 77, 149-150
deHaen Nonproprietary Name Index (NNI), 6-7, 8-9, 20-21, 40
deHaen services, 149-150
Deichmann, William B., 76
Deleted drugs, 10, 11, 13, 33
Dental preparations, 8, 9, 10
Dentistry, 29, 88
Department of Drugs, American Medical Association, 8
Department of Pharmaceutical Sciences, Pharmaceutical Society of Great Britain, 10
Departmental libraries, 99, 156
Derwent services, 151
Descriptors, 102, 109, 112, 116-118, 125-131, 133, 136, 138-139, 151, 175-176
Desktop Analysis Tool for the Common Data Base, 89
Devices, therapeutic, 10, 148
Dewey Decimal classification, 99, 101
DIALOG, 160
Dictionaries, 28, 79, 92, 94
Dictionaries, medical, 79
Dictionaries, multilingual, 94
Dictionaries, pharmaceutical, 28, 94
Diem, K., 95
Directories, 90, 93-94
Directory of Information Resources in

the United States. Biological Sciences, 90
Directory of Information Resources in the United States. General Toxicology, 90
Directory of Licensed Pharmacies, 93
Directory of Published Proceedings, 146
Disclosures, patent, 86
Diseases of the Kidney, 81
Diseases of the Liver and Biliary System, 81
Diseases of Medical Progress: A Study of Iatrogenic Disease, 76
Diseases and Physical Conditions, Alcoholism, Dentistry, Drugs and Narcotics Addiction, Smoking, and Vital and Health Statistics (Price List 51A), 88
Disinfection, Sterilization and Preservation, 69
Dispensatory (U.S.), 6-7, 8-9, 16, 20-21, 40
Dispensing of Medication, 69
"Disposal of Hazardous Wastes," 74
Dissertation Abstracts, 90, 146
Dissertation Abstracts International Retrospective Index, 90
DM: Disease-A-Month, 62
Documenta Geigy, 95
Documents collection, 98
Doerge, Robert F., 82
Doping and Sports, 132
Dorland's Illustrated Medical Dictionary, 79
Dosage, 6-7, 16
Dosage, pediatric, 9, 13, 16, 73
Dosage forms, 6, 8, 9, 13, 14, 15, 29, 32, 34, 72, 86
Dreisbach, Robert H., 75
Drug,
See also specific aspects, e.g. Drug interactions, See also Interactions
"Drug Abuse Control Amendments," 70
Drug Abuse Films, 79
Drug abuse materials, 77-79
Drug addiction, 88
Drug analysis, 9, 10, 11, 13, 15

Drug and Cosmetic Industry, 62
Drug Disposition and Pharmacokinetics — with a Consideration of Pharmacological and Clinical Relationships, 72
Drug Evaluations, AMA, 4, 6-7, 8-9, 16, 20-21, 23, 26-27, 40
Drug-Induced Diseases, 76
"Drug-Induced Modifications of Laboratory Test Values," 83
Drug Information Association, 63
Drug Information Bulletin, 63
Drug information centers, 46, 48, 96, 184-185
Drug Information Journal, 63
Drug information network, 184-185
Drug Information Services: Two Operational Models, 48
"Drug Information Sources" (Bloomfield), 28, 46
"Drug Information Sources" (Special Libraries Association), 28, 50
Drug information specialist, 96, 177-179
Drug Intelligence and Clinical Pharmacy, 59, 62, 64, 68
Drug interactions,
See also Interactions
Drug Interactions, 76
Drug Interactions (bimonthly), 77
Drug Interactions-1 and -2, 77, 114, 166
Drug Interactions — An Annotated Bibliography, 77
Drug Literature, 48, 65-66
Drug Literature Evaluation, Conference on, 179
Drug Literature Index, 134
"Drug Literature Utilization: Selection, Evaluation and Communication," 50
Drug products, definition, 32
Drug Research Reports, 62
Drug searching in BIOSIS, 136-138
Drug searching in Index Medicus, 129-131
Drug Topics, 14, 29, 61
Drug Topics Red Book, 6-7, 14-15, 19, 22-23, 29, 32, 33, 37, 38, 42, 168

Drug Trade News, 62
Drug Use in America: Problems in Perspective, 78
DRUGDOC, 134
Drugs,
　See also specific aspects, *e.g.*, Drug interactions, See also Interactions
Drugs, 63
Drugs, definition, 32
Drugs of Choice, 6-7, 8-9, 20-21, 29, 40
Drugs in Combination, 149
Drugs in Current Use and New Drugs, 6-7, 10-11, 20-21, 40
Drugs in Prospect, 149-150
Drugs in Research, 150
Drugs in Use, 149
Drugstore, 69, 85, 92, 93, 115, 167, 188
Drugstores, 88
Dulbecco, Renato, 81
Dunn, Donald A., 165, 166, 173

Economic poisons, 74-77
Economics, 65
Economics of future information handling, 165-166
Edge-notched cards, 181-182
Editorial manuals, 54-55
Editorials, 58
Education, continuing, 166, 172, 177
Education at home, 166
Educational Film Library Association, 79
Educational Resources Information Center (ERIC), 160
"Effects of Drugs on Clinical Laboratory Tests," 82
8 mm Film, 173
Eisen, Herman N., 81
"Electrocardiograms of the Month," 58
Elements, atomic weights, 11
Elkins, H. B., 75
Elsevier's Dictionary of Pharmaceutical Science and Techniques, in Five Languages, 94
EM *(Excerpta Medica)*, 113, 133-134, 160
Emergency room, 132

Encyclopedic treatises, 154-155
Endocrinology, 81
Endocrinology, 58
Engineering Index, 148
Environmental pollution, 143, 160
Environmental Protection Agency, 160
EP, 6-7, 10-11, 20-21, 28, 29, 30, 40
Epinephrine, 34
Epsom salt, 34
Equipment, 15, 93, 173
Equivalents, 6, 6-7, 28, 32, 34, 35, 89
ERIC (Educational Resources Information Center), 160
Ethical drugs, 9, 11, 13, 15, 31
Ethics, 65
European products, 8-9, 21
European Society for the Study of Drug Toxicity, 68
Evaluation of Drug Interactions, 76
Evaluation of drugs, 8, 10, 29, 68
Evaluation of literature, 56, 59, 85-86, 153, 178-180
Evaluation of searches, 111
Excerpta Medica (EM), 113, 133-134, 160
Executive Directory of the U.S. Pharmaceutical Industry, 93
Experiment station reports, 135
Experimental number,
　See Laboratory number
Expert Committee on Drug Dependence, WHO, 78
Extra Pharmacopoeia (Martindale) Incorporating Squire's Companion, 6-7, 10-11, 20-21, 28, 29, 30, 40

Facts and Comparisons, 6-7, 7, 10-11, 20-21, 29, 41
Faculty publications, 99
Falconer, Mary W., 40
FarmDoc, 151
Fate of Drugs in the Organism, 71
FDA, 12, 14, 15, 25, 26, 27, 34, 76, 85, 87, 149, 185
FDA Clinical Experience Abstracts, 148-149
FDA Drug Bulletin, 61
FDA Papers, 61

F-D-C Reports, 62
"Federal Food and Drugs Act," 25, 70
Federal Register, 27, 34
Federal Regulations, Code of, Title 21, 27
Federal Trade Commission, Bureau of Economics, 88
Federation of American Societies for Experimental Biology, 135
Fédération Internationale de Documentation, 148
Federation Proceedings, 135
Feed additives, 14, 22
Files, personal, 180-183
Files, subject, 180-183
Filing equipment and supplies, 93, 181
Filing rules, 102-103, 118-119, 129, 180-183
Films, 78-79, 172-173
Final Report, Project to Develop, Evaluate, and Demonstrate a Pilot Drug Information and Drug Therapy Analysis and Reporting System, University of Michigan Regional Drug Information Network, 48
Financial information, 93
First aid in poisoning, 6-7, 7, 74, 75
Flack, Herbert L., 190
Flack-King filing system, 181
Food and Drug Administration, 12, 14, 15, 25, 26, 27, 34, 76, 85, 87, 149, 185
Food, Drug, Cosmetic Law Reporter, 63
Foods, animal, 14, 22
Foreign code numbers, 36
Foreign drug handbooks, 9, 11, 13, 15, 28, 29, 30, 35
Foreign drugs, 9, 11, 13, 15, 21, 24, 28, 29, 30, 34, 35, 44, 46-51
Foreign-language journal articles, 112, 157, 176
Forman, Howard I., 91
Format aspects of drug handbooks, 37
Formula indexes, 13, 15, 21, 22, 23, 29, 35-36, 121, 123, 124
Formularies, hospital, 8, 27, 188

Formulas, structural, 11, 13, 15, 29, 35-36, 124, 151
Formulations, 6, 8, 9, 13, 14, 15, 29, 32, 34, 72, 86
Fortschritte der Medizinische Chemie, 57
Fragment searching, 122, 124, 151
Fragmentation index, 151
Francke, Donald E., 47, 73
Free and inexpensive material, 68, 86, 88
Free terms, 151
French names, 20
Fundamentals of Clinical Pharmacokinetics, 72
Fundamentals of Drug Metabolism and Disposition, 71
Fungi, 148
Fungicides (Handbook of Toxicology), 76
Furadantin®, 34
Furnishings, 93
Future, 164-192
Future technology, 175-176

Gaeke, Mary Ellen B., 181, 190
Gaeke, Richard F., 181, 190
Gaffin, Ben, and Associates, 91
Garbled prescriptions, 6
Garfield, Eugene, 66
General Pharmacology, 154
General Subject Index (CA), 116
Generic Index, Cumulated (BIOSIS), 141
Generic names, 14, 33, 34, 35, 116-117, 120, 131, 134
Geographic indexes, 131, 136
Georgia, University of, 158
Gerarde, Horace W., 76
Gestation periods, 15
Getting the original publication, 156
Gibaldi, Milo, 72
Gibberman, Val, 82
Gillette, J. R., 154
Gilman, A., 4, 7, 108
Ginsberg, Harold S., 81
Gisvold, Ole, 82
Gleason, Marion N., 74
Goldstein, Avram, 71

Goodale's Clinical Interpretation of Laboratory Tests, 82
Goodman and Gilman, 4, 71, 108
Goodman, L. S., 4, 71, 108
Gosselin, Robert E., 74
Gould Medical Dictionary, 79
Government documents, 68, 87-90, 98-99, 135, 146
Government Periodicals and Subscription Services (Price List 36), 88
Government Printing Office, 88-90
Government Reports Technical Announcements, 89
Government Research Announcements, 89
Government Research Index, 89, 146
GPO (Government Printing Office), 88-90
GRA, 89
Graa, Albert, 94
Greek alphabet, 13
"Green Sheet," 61
GRI, 89
Griffenhagen, George B., 31, 37, 41
Griffiths, Mary C., 42
GRTA, 89
Guide to Abstracting Services, Volume 1, Science, Technology, Medicine, Agriculture, 148
Guide to the Health Care Field, 93-94
Guide to the Literature of the Life Sciences, 54
Guide to the Use of the Excerpta Medica Abstract Journals, 133-134
Guide to the Vocabulary of Biological Literature, 138-139, 141-143, 180
Guides to secondary publications, 157
Gull, C. D., 143
Gupta, R. C., 17, 41
Gustafson, Carroll B., 69
Gustafson, Edward A., 40

Hair preparations, 10
Handbook of Analytical Toxicology, 75
Handbook of Basic Pharmacokinetics, 72
Handbook of Clinical Drug Data, 73
Handbook of Experimental Pharmacology, 154
Handbook of I.V. Additives Reviews, 73
Handbook of Medical Treatment, 80
Handbook of Non-Prescription Drugs, 6-7, 10-11, 20-21, 31, 33, 41
Handbook of Pharmacology, 71
Handbook of Poisoning, 75
Handbook of Toxicology, 76
Handbooks, drug, 4-40, 46-47
Handbooks, encyclopedic, 154-155
Handbooks, medical, 79-80
Handbücher, 154-155
Hansell, Dan N., 15
Hansten, Philip D., 76
HAPAB, 160
Harrison's Principles of Internal Medicine, 80
Hassan, William E., Jr., 69
Hawkins, Linda L., 31, 37, 41
Hayes, Edward N., 93
Hayes Druggists' Directory and Commercial Reference Book, 93
Health Aspects of Pesticides Abstract Bulletin (HAPAB), 160
Health Effects of Environmental Pollutants (HEEP), 143, 160
HEEP (Health Effects of Environmental Pollutants), 143, 160
Heffter-Heubner Handbuch der experimentellen Pharmakologie, 154
Heller, William M., 190
Hellums, Betty Ann, 46, 48
Henry, John Bernard, 82
Herxheimer, A., 76
Hierarchical lists, 127-128
Hierarchical searching, 127-128, 162
Highly specialized services, 148-151
Hirschman, Joseph L., 46
Hirtz, J., 71
Historical collections, 99
History of drugs, 6-7, 8, 9, 13, 17-18, 87, 109, 149-150
History of pharmacy, 50, 63, 69
History of Pharmacy, 69
HND, 6-7, 10-11, 20-21, 31, 33, 41
Hodge, Harold C., 74
Hofman, Frederick, G., 154
Holography, 175-176

Hopkins, Jenny, 28, 48, 82
Hospital Abstracts, 148
Hospital directories, 93-94
Hospital Emergency Room, 132
Hospital formularies, 8, 27, 188
Hospital Formulary Service, American, 6-7, 8-9, 16, 20-21, 27, 40, 180, 181, 183, 187-188
Hospital Literature Index, 148
Hospital Pharmacy, 62, 84
Hospital Pharmacy (Lippincott's), 62
Hospital pharmacy bibliography, 114
Hospital Pharmacy News, 84
Hospital Progress, 62
Hospital Tribune, 84, 85
Hospitals, 148, 167, 187
Hospitals, 62, 93
House organs, 64, 84-85
Household chemicals, 74
How to Find Out in Chemistry, 54
How to Find Out in Pharmacy, 46
How to find periodical titles of interest, 64-65
How to Promote Your Retail Pharmacy: A Guide to Publicity, Advertising, Promotion, 69
How to Use a Medical Library, 52
Hunnius, Curt, 94
Husa's Dispensing of Medication, 69
Husa's Pharmaceutical Dispensing, 69
Hypertension Bulletin (Hospital Tribune), 84
Hypertension; Diagnosis, Occurrence, and Prevention, 132

Identification, equivalent, 6, 6-7, 28, 32, 34, 35, 89
physical, 6-7, 10, 13, 15, 17
poisons, 6-7, 7, 10-11, 17, 22-23, 30, 41, 74, 75
Identification Guide for Tablets and Capsules, 6-7, 10-11, 17, 20-21, 41
Illinois Institute of Technology, 158
IM, 110, 113, 114, 125-133, 134, 149, 153, 166, 180
Importance of Fundamental Principles in Drug Evaluation, 68
Incompatibilities, physical, 6-7, 7, 16
Incompatibilities, therapeutic, 6-7, 7, 16, 76-77, 82-83, 110, 144-147
Index Chemicus, 124
"Index of Current Studies in Hospital Pharmacy," 90
Index to Dental Literature, 131, 132
Index Guide (CA), 116, 117, 120
Index Guide, Unlisted Drugs, 6-7, 14-15, 18, 23, 30, 36, 43
Index headings, 102, 109, 112, 116-118, 125-131, 133, 136, 138-139, 151, 175-176
Index Medicus, 110, 113, 114, 125-133, 134, 149, 153, 166, 180
Index of Mycology, 148
Index Nominum, 6-7, 10-11, 20-21, 41
Index of ring systems, 13, 121-122
Indexes to special materials, 146
Indexing services, 108, 112-151, 157-163
Indicators, 15
Industrial pharmacy periodicals, 62
Industrial toxicology, 74-75
Industry, pharmaceutical, 6, 6-7, 26, 60, 84-87, 93, 97, 151
INFORM, 160
Informatics, Inc., 134, 160
Information processing, 168
Information Services (CA), 122
Ingredients, 9, 13, 15, 74
Inke, Gabor, 52, 81
INN, 6-7, 10-11, 20-21, 34, 37, 41
Inorganic chemistry, 81-83
Input/output equipment, 168-170
Inquiry, 59
Insecticides, 10, 76, 89, 151
Insecticides (Handbook of Toxicology), 76
Inserts, package, 27, 84-85
Institute for Scientific Information, 124, 159
Institutional pharmacy periodicals, 61-62
"Institutions Holding Membership in the American Association of Colleges of Pharmacy," 93
"Integrated Health-Science Core Library for Physicians, Nurses and Allied Health Practitioners in Community Hospitals," 52, 80

Interactions, 6-7, 7, 16, 76-77, 82-83, 110, 144-147
Interactive searching, 162
"Interagency coordination in drug research and regulation," 48, 65-66
Interlibrary loan, 156-157
Internal medicine, 80
Internal Medicine (EM), 134
International Abstracts of Biological Sciences, 143
International Abstracts of Surgery, 148
International drug handbooks, 9, 11, 13, 15, 28, 29, 30, 35
International Encyclopaedia of Pharmacology, 154
International Federation of Pharmacy, 61
International Nonproprietary Names of Pharmaceutical Substances, 6-7, 10-11, 20-21, 34, 37, 41
International Nursing Index, 131, 132
International Pharmaceutical Abstracts, 65, 77, 113-114, 160, 166, 178, 180, 181
International Pharmacopeia, 6-7, 10-11, 13, 20-21, 41
International Standard Serial Number (ISSN), 189
International Union of Pharmacology, 155
International Union of Pure and Applied Chemistry (IUPAC), 35
Interpreting prescriptions, 6
Intravenous additives, 73
Introduction date, 9, 13, 17, 87, 109
Invasion of privacy, 167
Inverted files, 182
Investigational drugs, 14, 29, 30, 33, 150
  See also Products pending
Investigational number,
  See Laboratory number
Iowa Service, 150, 171
IPA Information System, 114
ISI (Institute for Scientific Information), 124, 159
Isolation and Identification of Drugs in Pharmaceuticals, Body Fluids and Postmortem Material, 6-7, 7, 10-11, 17, 22-23, 30, 41, 75
Isomers, 120, 128
Isoniazid, 86
Isselbacher, K., 80
ISSN (International Standard Serial Number), 189
IUPAC (International Union of Pure and Applied Chemistry), 35
I.V. additives, 73

Jackson, Elizabeth Christian, 46, 70, 81
JAMA, 58, 62
Japanese Journal of Pharmacology, 63
Japanese Pharmacological Society, 63
Japanese products, 8-9, 21
Jargon jungle, 31
Jasperson, H.-P., 41
Jawetz, Ernst, 80
Jeffrey, Louis P., 190
Jones, Tony E., 40
Journal of the American Chemical Society, 57
Journal of the American Dental Association, 9
Journal of the American Medical Association, 58, 62
Journal of the American Pharmaceutical Association, 61, 68, 93, 101
Journal of Bacteriology, 58
Journal of Clinical Pathology, 58
Journal of Clinical Pharmacology, 60
Journal clubs, 184
Journal of Experimental Medicine, 58
Journal of Health and Social Behavior, 59
Journal of Laboratory and Clinical Medicine, 63
Journal of Medicinal Chemistry, 58, 63
Journal Mondial de Pharmacie, 61
Journal of the National Cancer Institute, 58
Journal of Natural Products, 63
Journal of New Drugs, 60
Journal of Organic Chemistry, 57
Journal of Pediatrics, 58
Journal of Pharmaceutical Sciences,

59, 63, 72, 153
Journal of Pharmacology and Experimental Therapeutics, 63
Journal of Pharmacy and Pharmacology, 59, 63
Journal reference standards, 189
Journal of Urology, 58
Journals,
See Periodicals

Kabat, Hugh F., 83
Kalman, Sumner M., 71
Karczmar, Alexander George, 155
Kastrup, Erwin K., 41
Katz, Elihu, 91
Keeping up with the literature, 177-190
Keller, Bernard G., Jr., 69
Kepler, Judith A., 40
Kerker, Ann E., 54
Kern, K. R., 93
Keyword in Context (KWIC) indexing, 135-136
Keyword Subject Index (CA), 115
Keywords, 102, 109, 112, 116-118, 125-131, 133, 136, 138-139, 151 175-176
Kidney disease, 81
Kind of drug, 31-33
Kind of name, 27, 33-36
King, Charles M., Jr., 48, 190
Knapp, David A., 31, 37
Knoben, James E., 73
Kofoed, J., 17, 41
Krantz and Carr's Pharmacologic Principles of Medical Practice, 71
Kremers and Urdang's History of Pharmacy, 69
Krupp, Marcus A., 79, 80
KWIC (Keyword in Context) indexing, 135-136

L, 36
LA, 36
Labeled pharmaceuticals, 148
Laboratory numbers, 13, 15, 20, 22, 23, 30, 36
Laboratory tests, effect of drugs on, 11, 76-77, 82-83

La Du, Bert N., 71
Lamy, Peter P., 174
Lancet, 62
Lasagna, L., 155
Laser beams, 175
Lasslo, Andrew, 66
Latin American drugs, 24
Latin names, 11, 20, 37
Law for the Pharmacy Student, 69
Lawrence, Carl A., 69
Layman, 70, 173
Leadership, 191-192
Leake, Chauncey, 153
Learning Directory, 173
Legal System and Drug Control, 78
Legend drugs, 9, 11, 13, 15, 31
Legislation, 25-27, 69-70
Leith, Emmett N., 176
Lentner, C., 95
Letters to the editor, 58, 135
Level of effort in searching, 104-105
Levinson, Samuel Azor, 82
Lewis, Arthur J., 41
Lexikon für Apothekenpraxis in sieben Sprachen, 94
Libraries, 77, 96-103, 157-158, 184, 185
Library catalog, 98, 101-103
Library collection, 98-99
Library of Congress classification, 99, 100
Library of Congress Science and Technology Division, National Referral Center, 90
Library guides, 98, 99
Library studies of periodical use, 64
Licensing, patent, 87
Licensing, pharmacy, 93
Lilly, Eli & Company, 36, 84
Lilly Digest, A Survey of Community Pharmacy Operations, 85
Lippincott's Hospital Pharmacy, 62
"List of Most Frequently Recommended Medical Textbooks," 52
"Literature" (Wilson, C. O.), 50
Literature of Chemical Technology, 54
"Literature of Pharmaceutical and Medicinal Chemistry," 55

"Literature of Pharmacognosy and Medicinal Chemistry," 46
Literature Searches (MEDLARS), 132
Liver disease, 81
Lloydia, 63
Loan requests, 156-157
Local association journals, 60
Lockheed Information Retrieval Systems, 160
Loeb, Robert F., 80
Logic, computer search, 161
Look-alike prescriptions, 6
Looseleaf services, 39
Lowenthal, Werner, 174

Mac,
  See also Mc
MacFate, Robert P., 82
Macromolecular chemistry, 115
Magnesium sulfate, 34
Magnetic tape typewriters, 169
Main headings (*IM*), 125-131
Major descriptors (*IM*), 125-131
Mandel, H. George, 71
Mann, Michael, 88
Manual of Analytical Toxicology, 75
Manual to the Literature of Pharmacy, 46
Manual of Medical Therapeutics, 79
Manufacturers, 6, 6-7, 26, 60, 84-87, 93, 97, 151
Manufacturers' codes,
  See Code numbers
"Manufacturers of Hospital Pharmacy Equipment and Supplies," 93
Manufacturers' literature, 84-86
Manufacturing Chemist's Association, 74
Marihuana, 152
Marihuana: A Signal of Misunderstanding, 77-78
Market availability, 6, 6-7
Marketing, 69
Marketing date, 9, 13, 17, 87, 109
Marler, E. E. J., 42
Martin, Eric W., 69
Martindale's Extra Pharmacopoeia, 6-7, 10-11, 20-21, 28, 29, 30, 40

Massachusetts Institute of Technology, 173
Massachusetts Medical Society, 62
Mathematical tables, 95
Maurice, Jewell, 91
Mc,
  See also Mac
McDermott, W., 80
McEvilla, Joseph D., 88
McKay, R. James, 80
McLaughlin, Curtis P., 91
Medical bibliographies, 52-53, 132, 153
Medical books, 79-81
Medical Care, 59
Medical Care Reviews, 59
Medical Clinics of North America, 62
Medical dictionaries, 79
Medical Letter on Drugs and Therapeutics, 6-7, 7, 10-11, 16, 22-23, 29, 41, 61, 65
Medical libraries, 52-53, 96-103, 157-158, 184, 185
Medical Library Assistance Act, 185
Medical Literature Analysis and Retrieval System (MEDLARS), 125-133, 160, 162, 166
Medical profile systems, 9, 38, 167, 188
Medical records, 167, 187
Medical secondary publications, 125-134
Medical specialty periodicals, 58
Medical Subject Headings (MeSH), 110, 125-131, 133, 180
Medical and Surgical Motion Pictures: A Catalog of Selected Films, 173
Medical Tribune, 85
Medical World News, 85
Medicinal chemistry, 46, 54-55, 82
Medicinal Chemistry, 82
Medi-Kwok Index, 146
MEDLARS, 125-133, 160, 162, 166
MEDLARS On-Line, 64-65, 89, 125, 127, 132-133, 134, 158, 159, 160, 162, 185
MEDLINE, 64-65, 89, 125, 127, 132-133, 134, 158, 159, 160, 162, 185
Meeting announcements, 146

Meeting papers, 135, 146
Meeting proceedings, 146
Meeting programs, 146
Mellon, M. G., 54, 87
Melmon, Kenneth L., 73, 179, 190
Memex, 165
Menduke, Hyman, 179, 189, 190
Menzel, Herbert, 91
Merck Index; an Encyclopedia of Chemicals and Drugs, 2, 6-7, 12-13, 16, 22-23, 28, 29, 32, 35, 36, 37, 41
Mergers, 9
Merritt, H. Houston, 81
MeSH, 110, 125-131, 133, 180
Metabolism, 6-7, 16, 71
Metals and their compounds, 154
Meyler, L., 4, 76
Meyler's Side Effects of Drugs, 4, 76
Michigan Regional Drug Information Network, 48
Microbiology, 81
Microbiology, 81
Microcards, 170
Microdantin®, 34
Microfiche services, 74, 150-151, 170-171
Microfilm readers, printers and supplies, 93, 170-171
Microform publications, 74, 114, 150, 151, 170-171, 192
Micro-opaques, 170
Microphotography, 170-171
Milbank Memorial Fund Quarterly, 59
Miller, Lloyd C., 33, 37
Minor descriptors, 125-126, 127, 133
Mitchell, Stoklosa J., 69
Mittelstaedt, Stanley G., 43
Modell, Walter, 29, 40
Modern Drug Encyclopedia and Therapeutic Index, 6-7, 12-13, 22-23, 29, 33, 41
Modern Drugs, 6-7, 12-13, 23, 29, 41
Modern Hospital, 62
Modern Inhalation Anesthetics, 154
Molecular formulas, 13, 15, 21, 22, 23, 29, 35-36, 121
Molecular Pharmacology, 63
Moll, Wilhelm, 52

Monographs, 67-83, 98
Morrelli, Howard F., 73, 190
Morton, Leslie T., 52
Moser, Robert H., 76
Motion Picture Library, 173
Motion Picture and Videotape Catalog, 173
Motion pictures, 78-79, 172-173
Mullins, Patricia Moynahan, 50
Multilingual dictionaries, 94
Multiplicity principle in searching, 109-110
Murphy, Henry T., 54
Musto, David F., 78
Mycology, 148
NAFAIS (National Federation of Abstracting and Indexing Services), 189
Names, 6, 13, 27-28, 33-36, 89, 117-118
See also Author's terminology, Subject headings, Subheadings
Naming and Indexing of Chemical Substances for Chemical Abstracts, 118
Narcotic addiction, 88
NARD Journal, 61
National Aeronautics and Space Administration, 160
National Agricultural Library's Cataloging and Indexing System, 160
National Association of Boards of Pharmacy, 93
National Association of Retail Druggists, 61, 69
National Audio-Visual Association, Inc., 173
National Cancer Institute, Journal, 58
National Center for Poison Information, Rocky Mountain Poison Center, 74
National Clearinghouse for Drug Abuse Information, 77, 78
National Clearinghouse for Poison Control Centers, 74
National Commission on Marihuana and Drug Abuse, 77-78
National Coordinating Council on Drug Education, 79

National Drug Code Directory, 187-188
National Drug Information Service Center, 184
National Federation of Abstracting and Indexing Services (NAFAIS), 189
National Formulary, 6-7, 12-13, 22-23, 25, 31, 32, 34, 42, 184
National Formulary of Unofficial Preparation, 25
National Institute of Education, 160
National Institutes of Health, 91
National Library of Medicine, 48, 65-66, 76, 77, 89, 90, 125, 132, 160, 180, 184
National Library of Medicine classification, 99-100
National Medical Audiovisual Center, 173
National Referral Center, 90
National Research Council, 76
National Technical Information Service, 89-90, 160
Natural language (author's terminology), 109, 138-139, 151, 176
Nature, 61
"Nature and Magnitude of the Drug Literature," 48, 65-66
Nebraska, University of, College of Medicine, 173
Negwer, 6-7, 12-13, 22-23, 29, 32, 36, 42
Negwer, Martin, 6-7, 12-13, 22, 23, 29, 32, 36, 42
Nelson, Gaylord, 91
Nelson, Waldo E., 80
Nemec, Dolores, 48, 68-70, 79, 82
Network for Continuing Medical Education, 173
Networks, 157-163, 184, 185
Neurology, 81
Neuropharmacology, 63
New chemical compounds, 124
New Drug Application, 87
New drugs, 11, 15, 21
 See also Investigational drugs, Products pending, Patents
New Drugs, Evaluated by the A.M.A. Council on Drugs, 6-7, 11, 12-13, 22-23, 26-27, 42
New England Journal of Medicine, 58, 60, 62
New names, 14, 33-34
New and Nonofficial Drugs, 23, 26
New and Nonofficial Remedies, 25-26, 184
New York State Journal of Medicine, 58, 60
Newcombe, H. B., 190
Newell, Frank W., 81
News, 57-58
Newsletters, 64
NF, 6-7, 12-13, 22-23, 25, 31, 32, 34, 42, 184
99+ Films on Drugs, 79
Nitrofurantoin, 34
NND, 23, 26
NNI, 6-7, 8-9, 20-21, 40
NNR, 25-26, 184
Nomenclature rules, 35, 117-118
Nonlegend drugs, 9, 11, 13, 15, 16, 31, 33, 88
"Nonofficial" sources, 25
Nonprescription drugs, 9, 11, 13, 15, 16, 31, 33, 88
Nonproprietary Name Index, deHaen, 6-7, 8-9, 20-21, 40
Nonproprietary names, 14, 33, 34, 35, 116-117, 120, 131, 134
Northern, Robert E., 95
Notari, Robert E., 72
"Notices of Research Projects," 91
NTIS, 89-90, 160
Nuclear Science Abstracts, 148
Numerical Patent Index (*CA*), 115, 121
Nurses, 8, 29

Official Gazette of the U.S. Patent Office, 87
Oil, Paint and Drug Reporter, 62
Oldenberg, Henry, 57
Older drugs, 9, 16
On-line search programs, 161-162
On-line services, 113, 114, 122, 132-133, 134, 143, 151, 159-163
Ophthalmology, 81

Ophthalmology: Principles and Concepts, 81
Optical scanning devices, 169
Oral contraceptives, 32
ORBIT, 159-160
Organic chemistry, 54-55, 81-83, 115, 151
Organische-chemische Arzneimittel und ihre Synonyma (eine internationale Übersicht), 6-7, 12-13, 22-23, 29, 32, 36, 42
Organisms, 136, 141-143
Organization, 105-107, 177-183, 191
Organization of the collection, 99-101
Orientation sessions, library, 98
Orthography of drug names, 34
Oslet, J., 46
Osol, Arthur, 40, 51
Over-the-counter drugs, 9, 11, 13, 15, 16, 31, 33, 88
Overdose, 6-7, 7, 17, 74, 75

Package inserts, 27, 84-85
Packages, 8, 12, 14, 29, 93, 148
Pamphlets, 68, 86, 88
Parker, Edwin B., 165, 166, 173
PAS (Professional Activity Study), 187
Pasztor, Magda, 28, 48, 82
Patent Concordance (*CA*), 115, 121
Patents, 17, 31, 34, 55, 86-87, 115, 121, 151
Patient profile systems, 9, 38, 167, 188
Patterns and Consequences of Drug Use, 78
Patterson, H. Robert, 40
PDR, 6-7, 12-13, 22-23, 26, 27, 28, 31, 33, 42, 85
Pearson, Robert E., 46, 48
Pediatric dosage, 9, 13, 16, 73
Pediatric Dosage Handbook, 73
Pediatric Therapy, 80
Pediatrics, 80-81
Pediatrics, 58
Pediatrics (EM), 133
Peek-a-boo cards, 181-182
Peer review, periodical articles, 59
Penchansky, Roy, 91
Pending products, 13, 23, 29

See also Investigational drugs
Penicillin G and salts, 34
Periodical advertising, 60-61
Periodical articles, number, 64-66
Periodical contents lists, 64-65, 178
Periodical editing, 59-61
Periodical selection, 64-65
Periodicals, 46-55, 57-66, 67, 98, 101
Periodicals, analytical pharmacy, 63
Periodicals, business, 148
Periodicals, chemical, 54-55, 57-58, 62-63, 65
Periodicals, clinical chemistry, 63
Periodicals, clinical pharmacy, 62
Periodicals, community pharmacy, 61
Periodicals, government, 88
Periodicals, industrial pharmacy, 62
Periodicals, institutional pharmacy, 61-62
Periodicals, medical specialty, 58
Periodicals, pharmaceutical industry, 64, 84-85
Periodicals, pharmacology, 62-63
Periodicals, pharmacy, 46-50, 59, 61-63
Periodicals, physical pharmacy, 62-63
Periodicals, preclinical, 58
Periodicals, regional, state, and local, 60
Periodicals, research pharmacy, 62-63
Periodicals, social science, 59, 65
Permuted Subject Index (*SCI*), 146-147
Permuted title index, 135, 146-147
Permuterm Subject Index, (*SCI*), 146-147
Pernarowski, M., 72
Perrier, Donald, 72
Personal collections, 6-7, 38-44, 50, 64-65, 67-68, 85-86, 88, 153, 178-183
Personal files, 180-183
Perspectives in Clinical Pharmacy, 47, 73
PESTAB, 160
PestDoc, 151
Pesticides, 10, 89, 151
Pesticides Abstracts, 160
Petersdorf, R., 80
Pharmaceutic aids, 13, 15

Pharmaceutical Abstracts (APA), 114-115
Pharmaceutical Abstracts (Texas), 115
Pharmaceutical associations, 93, 177, 184, 186
Pharmaceutical Calculations, 69
Pharmaceutical chemistry periodicals, 62-63
Pharmaceutical company bibliographies, 84-86
Pharmaceutical dictionaries, 28, 94
Pharmaceutical Dispensing, 69
Pharmaceutical Division, Special Libraries Association, 14, 30, 86
Pharmaceutical Handbook, incorporating the Pharmaceutical Pocket Book, 94
Pharmaceutical industry, 6, 6-7, 26, 60, 84-87, 93, 97, 151
Pharmaceutical industry periodicals, 64, 84-85
Pharmaceutical Manufacturers Association, 35, 158, 160, 172
Pharmaceutical Marketing, 69
"Pharmaceutical Sciences: Literature Review of Pharmaceutics," 72, 153
Pharmaceutical Society of Great Britain, 10, 28, 40, 63, 94
Pharmaceutical technology, 94, 114
"Pharmacist as a Book Collector," 50
Pharmacist's Reference Shelf, 48, 68-70, 79
Pharmacognosy, 46
Pharmacognosy, 69
Pharmacokinetics, 72
Pharmacokinetics, 72
Pharmacologic Principles of Medical Practice, 71
Pharmacological Basis of Therapeutics, 4, 71, 108
Pharmacological and Chemical Synonyms; a Collection of Names of Drugs and Other Compounds Drawn from the Medical Literature of the World, 6-7, 12-13, 22-23, 28, 34, 42
Pharmacological Reviews, 63, 152
Pharmacology, 6-7, 16, 70-73, 134, 138, 143, 151, 154-155
Pharmacology books, 70-73
Pharmacology periodicals, 62-63
Pharmacology for the Physician, 62
Pharmacology and Toxicology (EM), 133
Pharmacopeia of the United States of America (The United States Pharmacopeia), 6-7, 14-15, 22-23, 24, 25, 31, 32, 33, 34, 42, 138, 184
Pharmacy, clinical, 70, 73
Pharmacy administration, 115
Pharmacy books, 68-70
Pharmacy colleges, 46, 50, 70, 93
Pharmacy in History, 63
Pharmacy News, 84
Pharmacy periodicals, 46-50, 59, 61-63
Pharmacy scope, 45, 56
Pharmacy secondary publications, 113-115, 148-151
Pharmacy Times, 61
"Pharmacy — Today and Tomorrow," 93
Pharmazeutisches Wörterbuch, 94
pharmIndex, 6-7, 12-13, 22-23, 29, 31, 42
Philips Roxane Laboratories, Inc., 84
Phillips, George L., 48
Philosophical Transactions of the Royal Society, 57
Photographic transmission, 171
Physical chemistry, 115
Physical identification, 6-7, 10, 13, 15, 17
Physical incompatibilities, 6-7, 7, 16
Physical pharmacy periodicals, 62-63
Physical properties, 6-7, 17, 75, 95
Physicians' Desk Reference, 6-7, 12-13, 22-23, 26, 27, 28, 31, 33, 42, 85
Physician's Handbook, 80
Physiological Basis of Medical Practice, 79
Physiological Pharmacology, A Comprehensive Treatise, 154
"Pink Sheet," 62
Pittsburgh, University of, 158
Poisindex, Inc., 74
Poison Cards, 74

Poison Detection in Human Organs, 75
Poison information and control centers, 9, 74
Poisoning — Toxicology-Symptoms-Treatments, 75
Poisonous substances, 6-7, 7, 17, 74-77
"Popular and Semi-Popular Reading List on Drugs," 70
Postaner, L. C., 82
Pratt, Robertson, 40
Preclinical periodicals, 58
Preliminary 8 mm Film Project Report and Listing of 8 mm Films, 173
Prescription drugs, 9, 11, 13, 15, 31
Prescription Pharmacy, 69
Prescription writing, 9, 169
Prescriptions, interpreting, 6
President's (de Bakey) Commission on Heart Disease, Cancer and Stroke, 184-185
Price of drugs, 6, 6-7, 29
Price of handbooks, 40-43, 44
Price index, 7, 10-11, 29
Price Lists (GPO), 88
Price of searches, 162-163, 165-166
Primary sources, 45-95
Principles of Biochemistry, 81
Principles of Drug Action. The Basis of Pharmacology, 71
Principles of Internal Medicine, 80
Privacy, 167
Problems of Species Difference and Statistics in Toxicology, 68
Proceedings in Print, 146
Proceedings of the Royal Society of Medicine, 58
Proceedings of the Society of Experimental Biology and Medicine, 58
"Procurement of Patents," 87
Product comparison, 10-11
Product Management, for the Drug, Cosmetic and Allied Industries, 62
Products pending, 13, 23, 29
See also Investigational drugs
Professional Activity Study (PAS), 187
Profiles, interest, 64-65, 157-158, 159, 163, 192
Profiles, patients', 9, 38, 167, 188
Profitable Drugstore Management, 69
Progress in Drug Research, 153
Progress Reviews, 152-154
Project to Develop, Evaluate, and Demonstrate a Pilot Drug Information and Drug Therapy Analysis and Reporting System, University of Michigan Regional Drug Information Network, 48
Project Intrex, 173
Promotion, 69
Prompt publication of journal articles, 59-60
Properties, physical and chemical, 6-7, 17, 75, 95
Proprietary rights, 33
Provost, George P., 60, 65
Psychological Abstracts, 160
Psychopharmacology Abstracts, 148
Public Health, Social Medicine and Hygiene (EM), 133
Public Law 89-239, 184
Public Law 89-291, 185
Public libraries, 77
Publication in parts (*EM*), 133
Publicity, 69
Purposes of drug handbooks, 8, 10, 12, 14, 28-30

Qualifiers, 128-129
Quality Control, 72
Quality control of a search, 111
Quantity of publication, 64-66

R, 36
Radioactive pharmaceuticals, 148
Ratcliff, Wendy W., 52, 80
Rational Drug Therapy, 62
Reactions, chemical, 13, 124
Reading, 178
Reagents, 11, 13, 15
Recent advances reviews, 152-154
RECON, 160
Record keeping, 105-107, 177-183
Recurring bibliographies (MEDLARS), 132
Red Book, 6-7, 14-15, 19, 22-23, 29,

32, 33, 37, 38, 42, 168
Reference collection, 98
Reference Manual on Hospital Pharmacy, 95
Reference substances, 11
References found records, 107
References to other sources, in drug handbooks, 6-7
Regional association journals, 60
Regional drug information centers, 184-185
Regional Medical Libraries, 158, 185
Regional Medical Programs, 184-185
Registry Handbook-Name Section, 122
Registry number index, 122
Registry numbers, 15, 23, 89, 122
Regulatory agencies, 9, 13, 24-28
Reid, W. Malcolm, 54
Reilly, Mary Jo, 50, 189, 190
Remington's Pharmaceutical Sciences, 51, 68
Reports, technical, 89
Reprints, 180-183, 192
Research drugs, 35, 149-150
Research Grants Index, 91
Research pharmacy periodicals, 62-63
Research studies, 90-91
Research toxicology, 76
Reserve reading room, 98
Resources beyond the local library, 156-163
Retail pharmacy, 69, 85, 92, 93, 115, 167, 188
"Review of Reviews," 153
Reviews of the literature, 57-58, 64-65, 72, 108, 121, 152-154
Ring systems index, 13, 121-122
RingDoc, 151
Ritschel, W. A., 72
Ro, 36
Roche Laboratories, 36, 173
Rocky Mountain Poison Center, 74
Roe, Robert, 80
Root, Walter S., 154
Rosenfeld, Michael G., 79
Rotated molecular formula index, 124
Rotated title index, 135-136

Rotated Wiswesser Line Notation, 124
Rotenberg, Gerald N., 40
"Rounds" presentations, 58
Royal Society, Philosophical Transactions, 57
Royal Society of Medicine, Proceedings, 58
Russian alphabet, 13

Safety Guides, 74
Sales statistics, 85, 88, 92
Salts of drugs, 119-120, 128
Sandford, A. H., 82
Sandoz-Warner, Inc., Basel, Switzerland, 84
Sax, N. Irving, 74
Scandinavian Journal of Clinical and Laboratory Investigation, 63
Scandinavian Society for Clinical Chemistry and Clinical Physiology, 63
Scheu, John D., 15
Schipma, Peter B., 189, 190
Schools of pharmacy, 46, 50, 70, 93
SCI (Science Citation Index), 109, 124, 144-147
Science, 61
Science Citation Index, 109, 124, 144-147
Scientific American, 61
Scientific Meetings, 146
Scientific Tables, 95
Scope and coverage of drug handbooks, 30
Scope of pharmacy, 45, 56
SDC (System Development Corporation), 159-160
SDI, 64-65, 157-158, 159, 163, 192
SDILINE, 132
Seal of Acceptance, AMA, 26
Search costs, 162-163
Search strategy, 107-111, 162
Searches, customized, 114, 143, 157-158, 159, 162-163
Searching the literature, 104-111, 161-162
Searching on-line, 161-162
Secondary publications, 64-65, 108,

112-151, 157-163
Section on Pharmacology and Biochemistry, Academy of Pharmaceutical Sciences, 68
See cross references, 126
See related cross references, 126
See under cross references, 126-127
Selected Government Publications, 88
"Selected List of Books and Journals for the Small Medical Library," 52, 80
"Selected List of Journals for the Small Medical Library: A Comparative Analysis," 52
Selection of literature sources in searching, 107-111
Selective dissemination of information, 64-65, 157-158, 159, 163, 192
Self-medication, 31
Senate Committee on Government Operations, Subcommittee on Reorganization and International Organization, 48, 65-66
Senate Select Committee on Small Business, Subcommittee on Monopoly, 88
Sewell, Winifred, 30, 48, 65-66, 83
Shafton, Allan L., 190
Sherlock, Sheila, 81
Sherrington, Andrew M., 91
Shirkey, Harry C., 73, 80
Short, Arthur, 42
Side effects,
See also Adverse reactions
Side Effects of Drugs: A Survey of Unwanted Effects of Drugs Reported in 1968-1971, 76
Siegelman, Stanley, 40
Single entities, 9, 11, 13, 31-32, 119-120
SKF, 36
Slides, 172
Small Business Administration, 88
Smith, Elbert G., 124
Smith, Mickey C., 31, 37, 69
Smith, Roger C., 54
Smith, Roger P., 74
Smith, William E., 73, 179
Smith, William M., 190

Smith Kline and French, 36, 84
Smithsonian Science Information Exchange, Inc., 90-91
Smoking, 88
Snowball search, 109, 152
Social Responses to Drug Use, 78
Social science periodicals, 59, 65
Social Work, 59
Société Suisse de Pharmacie, 10
Société de Technique Pharmaceutique, 71
Society of Experimental Biology and Medicine, Proceedings, 58
Society of Toxicology, 63
Solutions, 13, 15
Sonnedecker, Glenn, 50, 69
Sound-alike prescriptions, 6
Source Index (*SCI*), 146
Sources checked records, 105-107
Southeastern Michigan Hospital Council, 187
Southern Medical Journal, 60
Spanish names, 24
Special features of drug handbooks, 36-37
Special Interest Packages, Smithsonian Science Information Exchange, 91
Special Libraries Association, 14, 28, 30, 50, 86
Special subject secondary publications, 146-148
Specific compounds related to a single drug, 119
Specifications for the Quality Control of Pharmaceutical Preparations, 6-7, 10-11, 13, 20-21, 41
Specificity principle in searching, 110
Spelling of drug names, 34
Sports, 132
Sprowls, Joseph B., 69
Squibb, E. R., & Sons, 85
SSIE Science Newsletter, 91
Stanaszek, Walter F., 51, 73
Standardization, 95, 177, 186-189, 191, 192
  of literature data bases, 188-189
  of microforms, 170
Standardized vocabularies, 109, 116-

118, 125, 151
Standards for drugs, 10, 12, 13, 14, 24-28
Standards for names, 33-34
State association journals, 60
State laws, 69-70
Statistics, 85, 88, 92, 179
Stearns, Norman S., 52, 80, 81
Stecher, Paul G., 41
Stedman, Thomas L., 79
Stedman's Medical Dictionary, 79
Steinbichler, Evaline, 94
Stephenson, Hadley C., 43
Sterilization, 69, 94
Storage facilities, 93
Story of Health, 172
Strauss, Maurice B., 81
Structural formulas, 11, 13, 15, 29, 35-36, 124, 151
Style manuals, 54-55
Su, 36
Subheadings, 128-129
Subject files, 180-183
Subject heading definitions, 126-128
Subject headings, 102, 109, 112, 116-118, 125-131, 133, 136, 138-139, 151, 175-176
Subject Index (B.A.S.I.C.), 135-138
Subject reviews, 152-154
Subscriber response systems, 166
Substructure searching, 122, 124, 151
Summary of Major Findings, Final Report of the Task Force on Prescription Drugs, 92
Sundries, 10
Sunshine, Irving, 75
Superintendent of Documents, 88-90
Supplements to drug handbooks, 39
Supplies, 93
Surgery abstracts, 148
Surgery, Gynecology and Obstetrics, 148
Swarbrick, James, 72
Sweet, Norman J., 80
Swiss Pharmaceutical Society, 10
Symposia, 67, 68
"Symposium on a New Drug Compendium," 5
Synonyms, 6, 6-7, 28, 32, 34, 35, 89,
125-126, 138
System Development Corporation (SDC), 159-160

Table 1, 6-7
Table 2, 8-15
Table 3, 20-24
Table 4, 40-43
Table 5, 46-55
Tables of contents, 64-65, 178
Tape recorder, 172
Tariff and Taxation (Price List 37), 88
Task Force on Prescription Drugs, 92
Taube, Mortimer, 140, 143
Taxonomy indexes, 141-143
Taylor, Norman Burke, 79
Technical reports, 89
Technology, current, 165-174
Technology, future, 175-176
Technology, pharmaceutical, 94, 114
Tedeschi, D. H., 68
Tedeschi, R. E., 68
Telephone networks, 160-161, 169
Television, 172
Television, cable, 166
Television, closed circuit, 173
Teplitsky, Benjamin, 6
Terminals, cathode ray tube, 169
Terminals, computer, 160-161, 169, 176, 185, 192
Terms added to titles, 136-138
Tester, William, 150
Tests and assays, 9, 10, 11, 13, 15
Tetrahedron Letters, 58, 59
Texas, University, College of Pharmacy, 115
Textbook of Endocrinology, 81
Textbook of Medicine, 80
Textbook of Neurology, 81
Textbook of Organic Medicinal and Pharmaceutical Chemistry, 82
Textbook of Pediatrics, 80
Textbooks, 67-83, 98
Therapeutic devices, 10, 148
Therapeutic incompatibilities, 6-7, 7, 16, 76-77, 82-83, 110, 144-147
Therapeutic indications, 6-7, 16
Theses, 46, 90-91, 99, 146
Thesis Manual for Students in the

Pharmaceutical Sciences, 46
Third party claims, 9
Thomasson, C. Larry, 46, 50, 70, 81
Thorne, G. W., 80
Thudium, Vern F., 48
Tile and Till, 84
Time-limited reviews, 153
Time sharing, 161
Timour, John A., 52
Title enrichment, 136-138
Title indexes, 135-136, 146-147
Title pages, 64-65, 178
Todd, R. G., 94
Todd-Sandford Clinical Diagnosis by Laboratory Methods, 82
Toxicity, animal, 6-7, 7, 76
Toxicity Bibliography, 76, 132, 160, 166
Toxicology, 6-7, 7, 68, 70, 90, 154
Toxicology, analytical, 74, 75
Toxicology, industrial, 74-75
Toxicology and Applied Pharmacology, 63
Toxicology books, 74-77
Toxicology of Drugs and Chemicals, 76
Toxicology Information Program, National Library of Medicine, 90
Toxicology research, 76
TOXLINE, 114, 122, 143, 160, 185
Trade Name Cross Reference List, 114
Trade names, 32, 34, 35, 134
Trademark rights, 33
Trademarks Listed with the Pharmaceutical Manufacturers Association, 35
Tranquilizers (Handbook of Toxicology), 76
Translations, 112, 146, 157, 176
Translations Register-Index, 146, 157
Treatises, encyclopedic, 154-155
Treatment Manual for Acute Drug Abuse Emergencies, 78
Treatment and Rehabilitation (Drug Use in America), 78
Tree numbers, 127, 133
Tree Structures (*MeSH*), 125, 127-128

Triangle, Journal of Medical Science, 84
Tropical Diseases Bulletin, 148
Tuberculosis, 86
Tyler, Varro E., Jr., 69

UD, 6-7, 14-15, 18, 22-23, 29-30, 36, 43
Ultrafiche, 170
Unaccepted drugs (dental), 9
Unexpected sources of pharmacy information, 148
United States,
  See also U.S.
United States Adopted Names Council, 14, 33, 34, 35
United States Dispensatory, 6-7, 8-9, 16, 20-21, 40
United States Pharmacopeia, 6-7, 14-15, 22-23, 24, 25, 31, 32, 33, 34, 42, 138, 184
UNITERM indexing, 140-141
Universal drug compendium, 4-5
University of Alabama, 48
University of Georgia, 158
University of Nebraska College of Medicine, 173
University of Pittsburgh, 158
University search centers, 158-159
University of Texas College of Pharmacy, 115
Unlisted Drugs, 6-7, 14-15, 18, 22-23, 29-30, 36, 43
Unlisted Drugs Index Guide, 6-7, 14-15, 18, 23, 30, 36, 43
Unpublished Abstracts of Articles on Pharmaceutical Subjects, 115
Upatnieks, Juris, 176
Urdang, Georg, 69
Urology and Nephrology (EM), 133
U. S. Adopted Names, 6-7, 13, 14-15, 22-23, 27, 34, 35, 42
U. S. Dispensatory, 6-7, 8-9, 16, 20-21, 40
U. S. Food and Drug Administration, 12, 14, 15, 25, 26, 27, 34, 76, 85, 87, 149, 185
U. S. Government Printing Office, 88-90

U. S. Government Research and Development Reports, 89
U. S. Government Research and Development Reports Index, 89
U. S. Library of Congress, 90
U. S. National Institute of Education, 160
U. S. National Referral Center, 90
U. S. National Technical Information Service, 89-90, 160
U. S. Patent Office, 87
U. S. Pharmacopeia, 6-7, 14-15, 22-23, 24, 25, 31, 32, 33, 34, 42, 138, 184
U. S. Pharmacopeial Convention, 12, 14, 24-25, 34, 42
U. S. Senate. Hearings before the Subcommittee on Monopoly of the Select Committee on Small Business, 88
USAN Council, 14, 33, 34, 35
USAN and the USP Dictionary of Drug Names, 6-7, 13, 14-15, 22-23, 27, 34, 35, 42
USAN/USP-DDN, 6-7, 13, 14-15, 22-23, 27, 34, 35, 42
Usdin, E., 155
Use of Biological Literature, 54
Use of the Chemical Literature, 54
Use of literature sources in searching, 107-111
USP, 6-7, 14-15, 22-23, 24, 25, 31, 32, 33, 34, 42, 138, 184
Uvnäs, B., 155

Vaughan, Victor C., III, 80
Verification of loan requests, 156-157
VetDoc, 151
Veterinarians' Blue Book and Therapeutic Index; a Scientifically Descriptive Listing of Veterinary Drugs, Biologicals and Foods, and Feed Additives of American Manufacturers, 6-7, 14-15, 22-23, 29, 43
Veterinary drugs, 14-15, 28
Veterinary science, 151
Videotapes, 173
Virology, 58
Vital and health statistics, 88

Vitamins and Hormones, 153
Vocabularium Pharmaceuticum, 94
Vocabulary, standardized, 109, 116-118, 125, 151
Vocabulary browsing on-line, 161
Voice of the Pharmacist, 61
Voices-12/60, 172

Wachtel, Irma S., 143
Wagner, G., 190
Wagner, John G., 72
Walton, Charles A., 50
Washington University Department of Medicine, 79
Watanabe, Arthur S., 73
Way, E. Leong, 71
Webb, O. Lynn, 51, 73
Weber, David O., 79
Weekly Government Abstracts, 89
Weekly Pharmacy Reports, 61
Weights and measures, 11
Weil, B. H., 173
Weindling, Nelson, 92, 95
Welt, Louis G., 81
Western Journal of Medicine, 60
Westinghouse Learning Corporation, 173
White, Abraham, 81
"White Sheet," 62, 84
Whitney, Harvey A. K., Jr., 47, 73
WHO Chronicle, 21
Who's Who in America, 180
Widmann, Frances K., 82
Williams, Martha E., 190
Williams, Robert H., 81
Willis, J. H., 155
Wilson, Charles Owens, 40, 50, 82
Win, 36
Winthrop Laboratories, 36
Wintrobe, Maxwell M., 80
Wirephoto texts, 171
Wiswesser Line-Formula Chemical Notation, 124
Wiswesser Line Notation (WLN), 124
WLN (Wiswesser Line Notation), 124
Wood, D. N., 66
World Health Organization, 10, 41, 98

World Health Organization. Expert Committee on Drug Dependence. *Twentieth Report*, 78
"World List of Pharmacy Periodicals," 46
World Meetings, 146
Wyatt, H. V., 54

X, XR, and XU references, 126-127
Year Book of Drug Therapy, 153
Yearbooks, 152-154
Young, D. S., 82
Young, Marna Jo, 46

Zachert, Martha Jane K., 46, 50, 70, 81

DATE DUE